S0-AJB-705

Home Visits

A Return to the Classical Role of the Physician

Feb. 15, 2019

For Don,

I hope you enjoy this intimate portrait of care of the home visit patient. We so loved being with you this evening.

Fondly,

Alfred

Home Visits

A Return to the Classical Role of the Physician

Alfred E. Stillman MD, MACP

Radcliffe Publishing
Oxford • Seattle

Radcliffe Publishing Ltd
18 Marcham Road
Abingdon
Oxon OX14 1AA
United Kingdom

www.radcliffe-oxford.com
Electronic catalogue and worldwide online ordering facility.

© 2007 Alfred E. Stillman

Alfred E. Stillman has asserted his right under the Copyright, Designs and
Patents Act 1998 to be identified as author of this work.

All rights reserved. No part of this publication may be reproduced, stored in
a retrieval system or transmitted, in any form or by any means, electronic,
mechanical, photocopying, recording or otherwise without the prior
permission of the copyright owner.

British Library Cataloguing in Publication Data

A catalogue record for this book is available from the British Library.

ISBN-10: 1 84619 074 6
ISBN-13: 978 1 84619 074 2

Typeset by Advance Typesetting Ltd, Oxford, UK
Printed and bound by Biddles Ltd, King's Lynn, Norfolk, UK

Dedication

This book is dedicated to my wife, Paula, my constant source of inspiration and encouragement, who suggested that, after my career in gastroenterology seemed at an end, I go into geriatrics; to my mother, who guided me into medicine and lived to see me a happy geriatrician; to my father who, although unable to become a physician, always encouraged and supported my interest in medicine; and to my sons Norman and Michael, who respectively entered veterinary and allopathic medicine and who love medicine for all the right reasons.

However, this work is primarily dedicated to my patients, both living and dead, who have always reminded me why I love my profession.

Preface

I need to write this book to make people (the public and even my own colleagues in healthcare) aware of what I and a small group of geriatricians dedicated to home care practice do to take care of and bring comfort to a large group of anonymous people. These patients, due to physical ailments, cognitive disability or lack of social support, would not be able to obtain medical care today. This is not due to lack of insurance but because they simply cannot get to a doctor's office and the doctor can't or won't come to them.

In addition, I love my patients and their caregivers, not generically but individually. I want each of them to be remembered for the stoic heroism and even good humor that they exhibit every day under grinding burdens. I would like their lives to serve as an example to others and their plight to be a stimulus to our government and medical establishment to help relieve their predicament. This should be done not only for humanitarian reasons but also because these patients are a significant drain on health care financial resources, a drain that could be checked by judicious and timely application of home visit services.

I have also included a glossary of medical and administrative terms at the end of the book. This should ease understanding of the text by readers unfamiliar with medical terminology and prevent littering the text with explanations that can be more succinctly stated elsewhere.

Alfred E. Stillman
September 2006

About the Author

Alfred Stillman is a geriatrician whose practice is devoted primarily to the care of the elderly but also to morbidly obese and neurologically impaired patients all of whom are unable to easily leave their homes. He has always engaged in the private practice of medicine but has held numerous academic teaching appointments, authored many medical articles, and received prestigious awards as a private practitioner.

Dr Stillman practices in Philadelphia, PA but lives with his physician wife, Paula, in Bala Cynwyd, PA. They enjoy travel and theater but take special pride in their physician sons, their partners and their grandchildren.

Pre-history

I always wanted to be a doctor – that is, if you consider the beginning of "always" to be age four years. When little boys were fantasizing about being policemen or firemen and little girls were dreaming of being nurses or ballerinas, I was listening to stories, read to me by my mother, of the great physicians and medical innovators of history and setting my course toward joining their company.

Of course, the mid-1940s was a time when most Jewish mothers dreamt that their son would become a physician or that their daughter would marry (not become) one. The use of the singular for son and daughter is appropriate, because the Depression had rendered child rearing expensive and many families were only able to afford one child. I, like so many others born in my era, was an only child. Although my mother and father were each one of six siblings, there had been no physicians in my family. My parents centered great hopes on my medical career and planned for it methodically. My mother, a teacher, bought simple books such as *How Man Discovered His Body*, relating the stories of Andreas Vesalius, Anton van Leeuwenhook and William Harvey, and read them to me until I was able to read myself. My father, a pharmacist, brought back simple books on chemistry and read them with me. By age eight, I knew the periodic table of the elements. Although they oriented me towards scientific and particularly towards medical interests, my parents never neglected other facets of my development. My mother instilled in me a love of literature, especially poetry, while my father gave me a strong foundation in classical music.

When I entered the Bronx High School of Science at age twelve, I met a group of young, largely Jewish scholars who were also only children and who had been brought up in home environments similar to mine. They too, including the girls, aspired to become physicians. Bronx Science was just the place to nurture and shape the aspirations of these children and their families. My electives in high school were all in advanced biology and chemistry, and my foreign language was Latin. I purposely chose these to foster my understanding of medical material. (In the early 1950s, many knowledgeable people felt that Latin was a necessary prerequisite for the study of medicine). The biology club was one of the most popular extracurricular activities, and one that many students were eager to include in their résumés to bolster the appearance of their commitment to medicine. The atmosphere in Bronx Science was intensely competitive and not conducive to forming firm friendships other than those based on shared career aspirations. When I look back now on the list of my fellow graduates, I am not at all surprised to see the large number of physicians, and especially those who achieved eminence in medicine.

I entered Cornell University College of Arts and Sciences committed to using the next four years as a springboard to enter medical school. In the mid to late 1950s, this seemingly Machiavellian attitude was not uncommon. Many college students, conditioned by childhood in the Depression and World War Two, were specifically goal oriented and did not view college as a broadening experience and an end in itself as is so common among today's young adults. Accordingly, I majored in chemistry – at that time, the longest and one of the most difficult majors at Cornell – and gained Honors through research in physical and analytical chemistry. My extracurricular activities were few, but sufficient to demonstrate that I was a broad-minded candidate fit for medical school. In my senior year I was admitted to New York University School of Medicine.

At NYU, I again found my classmates to be mostly Jewish and even discovered several old Bronx Science acquaintances. Ten per cent of my entering class was female. The atmosphere was at last truly friendly and collegial. During my first year at medical school, in addition to the prescribed basic science courses, I became fascinated by cardiology and read extensively on the anatomy of the heart, electrocardiography and congestive heart failure. I also started a subscription to *Circulation*, which I faithfully read. During my final two years I became intensely interested in such a large number of potential medical and surgical specialties that my classmates good-naturedly laughed every time I expressed interest in yet another field. In those days, "the best and the brightest" entered general internal medicine. Our idols, about whom we still speak reverently at our medical school reunions, were the professors of internal medicine who were diagnostic "gods". Even in today's high-tech medical atmosphere, my classmates and I (and those physicians of our era) are amazed at how often these great clinicians achieved the correct diagnosis with only their discerning questions, practiced senses and enormous encyclopedic experience. Board examinations at that time existed for only a few internal medicine subspecialties, and subspecialty medicine had only just begun to attract the attention of young doctors as a career opportunity. It was at this time that I seriously considered ophthalmology as my future, until one of my classmates, Ruth Spritzer, commented that, if I did so, I would forget how to use a stethoscope. That one simple sledgehammer sentence changed my medical career forever. From then on, I would be devoted only to internal medicine. (Facility for aphorisms seemed to run in the Spritzer family. Ruth's physician father had once told me cryptically that "You will not be a good physician until you have filled a graveyard".) At graduation from medical school, our dean, Dr. S. Bernard Wortis, told us that "Medicine is a hard mistress and doesn't easily tolerate competition."

During my year of internship in internal medicine at Kings County Hospital–Downstate Medical Center in Brooklyn, New York, I worked the standard 36 out of 48 hours for a full year at a salary of $3200 per year. We house officers were too tired to socialize during our time off. I might go to a movie with another house officer on a night off, and spend an occasional free afternoon at the Brooklyn Museum or the Brooklyn Botanical Garden alone. Otherwise, I spent much of my limited spare time reading or sleeping.

During that first year, I discovered that an emaciated middle-aged man had achalasia. I worked with Dr. Edmund McNally, our program's gastroenterologist, who proved to be such a lovely, gentle man and a patient, inspiring teacher that I became enamored of gastroenterology (GI) and took my only elective month that year with him. At that time, before the proliferation of fiberoptic endoscopy, there were few certified gastroenter-ologists. Dr. McNally had trained under the renowned Dr. Franz Ingelfinger. During my last year of residency I obtained a GI fellowship under Dr. Norman Zamcheck at Boston City Hospital (BCH), to begin when I finished my required two-year tour of duty with the United States Public Health Service (USPHS).

After finishing my three years of internal medicine training, I entered the USPHS for two years and was stationed in New York City, Philadelphia, Alaska and Cincinnati. I started a subscription to several GI journals to ensure continued contact with my chosen field until the fellowship began. During my USPHS tour, I acquired a solid foundation in outpatient internal medicine and was also exposed in 1968 to the future face of socialized medicine. I recall that, in Cincinnati, our clinic had ordered our monthly quota of barium enemas when only 20 days in the month had passed. All of the patients who required a barium enema during the next 10 days would need to wait until the following month when it could be ordered again.

At BCH, "Dr. Z" taught me that "what makes a gastroenterologist is between his ears" – a lesson that I never forgot and which I still quote. This was admittedly at the beginning of the fiberoptic endoscopic era, when a gastroenterologist's knowledge of GI physiology was essential to his consultative effectiveness. Dr. Z also taught me to consider how I would conduct my defense before a Morbidity and Mortality Committee should a complication develop as the result of a procedure that I had either ordered or performed. The corollary of this axiom, extended to general internal medicine (and geriatrics), is to beware of ordering or even suggesting procedures that will have no obvious effect on the patient's welfare.

In Tucson, my first place of practice, I met Dr. Jack Marx, a local psychiatrist, who taught me to tune into the patient's *total* history – both social (in the broadest sense of the term) and medical – to achieve the greatest understanding of the patient. Since then, my consultative histories have always included a full patient résumé, including many events of which their primary care physicians (PCPs) had never been aware. My reports also included suggestions for remedying social as well as medical problems, and my opinion was sought by many internists and family practitioners. After practicing in Tucson for 13 years, my physician wife was offered a position as associate dean at a medical school, and my family and I moved to Worcester, Massachusetts, where I practiced GI for another 12 years.

After 27 years in consultative GI practice, I switched back to internal medicine and, within a year, to geriatrics. My wife and I had moved to Norfolk, Virginia in 1994 when she became the dean of Eastern Virginia Medical School, and I had been offered a position in GI on the medical school staff. Within a few months of our move, we both lost our positions and were unable to find jobs. In the mid-1990s, the medical establishment came to believe that there were too few generalists and too many subspecialists in practice. During that tumultuous time, many subspecialists lost their jobs and many newly trained young subspecialists could not find jobs. We moved to Philadelphia hoping that the large number of medical schools and teaching hospitals there would be advantageous for us.

At the age of 57, after a long, fruitless search for GI jobs and after a brief, unsatisfying stint in general internal medicine, I took a fellowship in geriatrics at the Albert Einstein Medical Center in Philadelphia. This was a calculated decision to ensure that I would never again have difficulty finding employment. It was common knowledge that the elderly were the fastest growing population segment in the United States, but despite this, American geriatric fellowships produced only 100 new geriatricians per year. I was by far the oldest house officer in the hospital, and was also older than all of my teachers. Some of my teachers could not break the habit of calling me "Dr. Stillman", although they called all other house officers by their first name. Nevertheless, a few of my teachers asked me to fill the role of house officers less than half my age but with none of my experience, and insisted that I draw patients' blood before morning rounds. My mentor in that program was Dr. Richard Grant, who taught me that, in contrast to most other specialties, success in geriatrics is measured by gain in or at least stabilization of *function*, and that practicing geriatrics often consists of "small victories" (for example, just a small gain in function might be enough to preserve a patient's independence). It was not necessary to address *every* deficit – only the vital ones.

During my geriatric fellowship, I found that I especially enjoyed doing home visits for elderly patients who were unable to leave their homes. Once again, my career-long love of talking to and getting to know people served me well. I was able to tailor my schedule to meet the needs of my patients, which usually involved seeing an average of five to eight patients per day in the community. After spending a year after my fellowship with the Albert Einstein Medical Center division of geriatrics, I joined Dr. Alan Berg in practice. Alan, an experienced and much admired geriatrician, had performed home visits on elderly patients unable to leave their homes to seek medical attention for many years. His expertise in dealing with the special, often exasperating problems of bringing medical and social help to these patients was vital in boosting my learning curve in the early years of our practice.

We have now practiced together for eight years and have added a geriatric nurse practitioner and a social worker to our practice. We see our patients only in their homes. We go to our office daily to answer messages, open mail and communicate with each other and our nurse practitioner, social worker and secretaries about the previous day's events and about puzzling problems. We never see patients in our office – our clinical work is performed in the community. We see almost all of the patients who are referred to us, provided that they live in our established geographical area. Our patients are referred to us by social agencies such as the Philadelphia Corporation for Aging (PCA), visiting nurse organizations, hospital discharge planners, elder day care centers and private physicians who realize that they no longer have the time to do justice to their homebound patients.

At this point, I would like to draw attention to the PCA, which figures prominently in many episodes in this book and in my daily practice. The federal government has mandated that each county in the United States must have an organization for the purpose of disbursing funds, dispatching personnel and dispensing information to ease the lot of our elderly poor. The PCA is a bulwark behind my practice and patients. They and their counselors are always ready and available to give advice about senior day programs, procure home health aides and nurses for needy elders, order extermination of bug-infested houses, extricate elders from dangerous living environments or attend to myriad other tasks. PCA and their associate organization, Adult Protective Services (APS), also investigate cases of suspected elder neglect or abuse, and are empowered to correct these situations.

When I first started to do home visits about 10 years ago, one of my patients was an elderly man who was hypertensive and diabetic and who had had a previous stroke. He was confined to a wheelchair. His wife, who was relatively healthy, was his sole caregiver and also took care of their apartment. The couple lived in a basement apartment whose only daylight entered through two dirty transoms. My patient was unable to go outside because their house did not have an elevator and he could not mount the few steps from the basement level to the front door. One day, I received a frantic call from the husband. His wife had collapsed in their home and had died in front of him. I immediately called the APS and they did not disappoint me. Within one hour they had arrived on the scene and empathetically arranged for the wife's burial. Within a few more hours, they had also arranged for admission of the husband to a nursing home.

On another occasion, one of my severely demented women patients, who was being cared for by her slightly less demented brother, was in danger during an infernally hot Philadelphia summer because her brother had decided not to waste money by turning on the air conditioning or fans, although the family was well off financially. Once again, I called the PCA, who responded immediately and whisked both sister and brother off to a nursing home while arranging for guardianship for both of them.

I cannot praise the PCA and APS sufficiently. They have limited funds but use these judiciously to superb effect. We home-visit physicians and health-care-related colleagues could not do our job properly without them. Although most people have not heard of these agencies or had occasion to need their services, I know that they are one of the best bargains we get for our tax dollar.

Although 90% of our patients are in the geriatric age group, about 10% are middle-aged or young adults. These individuals are either morbidly obese or have severe neuromuscular disease. Their homebound state and medical and social needs are just as implacable as those of our most disadvantaged elderly patients.

Geriatric and Other Types of Home Visits

Geriatrics is the branch of medicine that deals with the care of the elderly – in our society, commonly meant to be people over 65 years of age. Of course, we all know people aged 90 who are vital, stimulating and active, and others aged 55 who have lost interest in life's pleasures. The beginning of the geriatric age group probably relates to the classic age of retirement, although people may now work well beyond 65.

Geriatrics differs from most other medical disciplines in that it is a *functionally* oriented specialty. The geriatrician is the head of a team consisting of nurses, physical, occupational and speech therapists, social workers, medical equipment specialists, hospice workers and a host of like-minded home-care-oriented clinicians, including podiatrists, optometrists, audiologists, psychiatrists and dentists. *The team's objective is to maximize patients' independence on their own home turf for as long as possible.* This can best be accomplished by knowing each patient's individual home environment. During the home visit, the geriatrician faces a constant stimulating challenge to pit his knowledge and experience against a patient's symptoms and psychosocial problems without the easy and immediate access to and comforting convenience of consultation and laboratory or imaging facilities.

Within the past seven years, there has been a resurgence of applications among young physicians for positions as geriatric fellows. This has probably been due to a combination of two factors – first, the belated realization among many that our population is indeed aging and that the geriatric age group is the fastest growing sector, and secondly, the extraordinary and unique step taken by the American Board of Internal Medicine (ABIM) in *lowering* the number of years required for a geriatric fellowship from two to just one. As a result, a new generation of young physicians is entering practice with particular knowledge of the elderly and their special problems. Even if these doctors do not confine themselves to geriatric practice, their knowledge of and empathy with the geriatric population will certainly serve them and their patients in good stead.

However, even recent graduates of geriatric programs may not have a solid foundation in the care of the homebound. To be sure, all geriatric programs are required by the ABIM to expose their fellows to home care patients, but this is not strongly emphasized by most programs, probably because these patients are highly labor-intensive and offer little financial recompense, especially if they are poor and are insured by Medicaid or by Medicaid health maintenance organizations (HMOs).

The *elderly homebound* are a distinct subset within the geriatric population. For them, old age is not an anticipated rainbow's end after a life of work and family rearing, but rather it is a time of unabated loss as physical stamina and mental function implacably deteriorate, family and friends die, and even personal identity weakens during retirement or job loss. This is a time of dependency and loneliness for many formerly independent and gregarious people. Many older citizens will retreat into their homes because they are physically disabled (e.g. due to stroke, amputation, arthritis, heart failure, chronic lung disease, etc.) cognitively or emotionally disabled (e.g. due to dementia or depression), or afraid to socialize (due to fear or embarrassment of falling, incontinence or hearing or visual impairment), or because they are too far from or too infirm to use public transportation or do not have caregivers or friends to transport them. These patients cannot or will not leave their homes, often labor under a far greater chronic disease burden than ambulatory patients, and are a significantly medically neglected segment of our society.

Our practice consists of patients who, if not seen by us, would be largely seen only in an emergency room or hospital setting. It is not cost-effective for physicians practicing in an outpatient setting to disrupt their office routine for the 90–120 minutes that it might take to travel to and from the patient's house, perform the evaluation and submit the appropriate orders. It is much easier for the physician to order an ambulance to take the patient to the nearest emergency room, and it also allows the doctor to feel that they have "done the right thing" by having his patient seen in a high-tech academic or tertiary care center.

The vast majority of homebound patients' calls can be answered over the phone (as with any other patient), but only if that patient is already well known to the physician. A severe strain is placed on our health care dollar reserve by unnecessarily diverting resources to intensive evaluations of minor problems. Also, many small problems of the homebound, if caught early by an experienced physician who knows their patient, can be prevented from mushrooming into a major problem that will eventually require hospitalization. The PCP feels understandably nervous dealing with these patients (often capitated), whom he may not have actually seen for years. In addition, these patients, if injected into a busy ambulatory waiting room on a stretcher, might disrupt the office routine or patient flow either because of their potentially odd behavior or because their stretcher may take up too much room.

This group of complex, elderly, homebound patients with a significant chronic disease burden should be optimally handled by senior physicians devoted exclusively to home care practice working with geriatric nurse practitioners and social workers who know the patients and their backgrounds intimately and who have a good understanding of community support resources. These patients can be efficiently, thoroughly and unhurriedly evaluated in their homes, where we can:

- perform a complete history and physical examinations
- arrange for on-site visits from laboratories and respiratory, electrocardiographic and imaging companies (we can obtain ultrasound, echocardiographic and Doppler evaluations routinely at home)
- perform environmental assessments
- evaluate the patient's financial status
- examine refrigerators and cupboards for food type and availability as well as for alcoholic beverages
- inspect the patient's home for cleanliness
- look for and assess the need for safety devices on stairs, in bathrooms, etc.
- evaluate lighting or obstructing or dangerously placed objects
- obtain in-house consultations and medical services (already noted above)
- meet the family and caregivers
- develop a degree of intimacy and trust with these people, which would take a far longer time to achieve in an ambulatory setting
- assess the degree of involvement of the family and caregivers in care and relationship with the patient
- assess their personalities and availability, and determine who the major players are
- determine whether advance directives exist. Advance directives are usually living wills or individuals with durable power of

attorney who ensure that the patient's welfare is maintained should they no longer be able to make decisions for themselves. If they don't exist, we discuss the types of advance directives with the appropriate individuals

- determine the possible existence of elder abuse or neglect
- determine the emotional and physical stamina of the primary caregiver, and marshal community and other resources to ensure that this person has the support necessary to continue his or her function.

Home visits sound quaint – a practice from a bygone era, treasured in memory but regarded as substandard in this medically high-tech age. And yet I recall my pediatrician of more than 60 years ago, Dr. Barenberg, coming into our home late at night and worshiped by my educated parents. I can still recall the comforting feel of his hands on my face and chest, his always impeccable dress, and the faintly medicinal odor that hung around him. His confidence and comforting assurance when he spoke to my concerned parents were palpable in our small bedroom. Many doctors have examined me since then, but my memory of this earliest encounter has lasted the longest, is indelible and is the fondest of all these memories.

The memory of Dr. Barenberg reminds me of Luke Fildes' famous painting, *The Doctor*. The doctor is depicted in a solitary and lonely struggle to understand a little girl's illness and save her life. He is well dressed and wears an expensive ring – out of keeping with the poverty-stricken appearance of the home. The scene is set late at night. A single lamp illuminates the doctor, silent in intense thought, and his pale patient who is stretched across two chairs cushioned by pillows and appears very ill and out of touch with her surroundings. The figures of the anguished parents in the dark background are almost sensed rather than seen. Although we now have more knowledge and resources available to us than did this heroic physician, his spirit lives on in any doctor who enters a home for the benefit of his patient.

In my present practice, I feel the same devotion and respect from my patients. They offer me food and beverages on arrival, give me small tokens on special occasions, ask about my wife, children and grandchildren, remark on my appearance and always give me juice when I appear to be hypoglycemic (I have insulin-dependent diabetes).

Home visits are an especially *intimate* method of knowing a patient and his or her family. I am invited into the patient's home as a guest to witness their financial status, interpersonal relationships with relatives and caregivers, cleanliness, and food supplies, none of which are easily discernible by or volunteered to the physician who sees their patients in less familiar settings. Home visits show the doctor how his hospitalized or ambulatory office patient was "made." *The doctor must earn that trust.* He must be able to judge clinical situations rapidly and accurately without immediate recourse to laboratory, imaging, EKG or consults, and have the knowledge and capability to treat most conditions at home while knowing the limits of his capabilities. He must also deliver his care non-judgmentally and sympathetically. This ability is strengthened not only by previous experience with and knowledge of each individual patient's medical history, but also by first-hand experience of their living environment, interactions with caregivers (if any) and support systems. I believe that home visits should preferably be performed by seasoned, experienced clinicians who are confident in their ability to act independently.

Most of our patients are impoverished and live either in black ghettos or in senior apartment houses. Some live in older attached houses. A few live in sumptuous apartments or houses and are well off. Our poor patients are medically insured by Medicare and/or Medicaid, and only a few of our patients have expensive, comprehensive insurance plans. Many of our patients are malnourished because they can't afford food, have no one to buy food for them (if they are unable to leave their home), or have no one to prepare a meal for them (if they are physically or cognitively unable to do so). Many subsist on frozen meals delivered by subsidized charitable organizations. We often cannot order such meals with specified sodium and carbohydrate content. Even our poorest patients make every attempt to keep their homes neat and clean. Some have vermin-infested homes, but this is often beyond their control. The patients usually bathe themselves or are bathed by their caregivers before our arrival. Even the oldest women usually have a bottle of toilet water or cologne on their bathroom counter.

I would now like to introduce you to some of my patients, both living and deceased, whose company I have so enjoyed and whose daily struggles have never been far from my thoughts.

It is much more important to know what sort of patient has a disease than what sort of disease the patient has.

Sir William Osler

The Patient Posing a Moral or Ethical Dilemma

When Jack died, I felt combined sadness and relief. I usually feel sad when one of my patients dies. After all, I have generally cared for them for at least one (and often up to seven) years, and one can't easily do that without losing some objectivity and regarding them as friends, too. I had been Jack's physician for two and a half years. In his case, I was relieved because I had known from the start of his final weeks that he would die shortly and that he was going through mental and emotional as well as medically symptomatic anguish.

Jack was 79 years old and blind due to glaucoma. He lived alone in a two-story house and, like many of my blind but mobile patients, was able to confidently navigate around both floors without falling or colliding into objects. He was well spoken, with only a high-school education, and was the proud father of five children. Their photographs and records of their achievements adorned the walls in place of the expected paintings and other memorabilia. The children had all graduated from college, and one was a physician in another state. He told me that they all phoned him and that at least his daughter often visited him. I knew this was true because his physician son had called me several times before his dad's final illness to check on his condition. Jack depended on a neighborhood storekeeper to bring his lunch daily. He could prepare his own simple breakfast, while his supper, baths, errands and other creature comforts were provided by a home health aide furnished by the PCA. Jack's medications were carefully lined up on the table next to his favorite chair, and he took them without any assistance. Although he rarely went out of doors and never without help, in his own home he was king and proud of his limited independence.

Until the last month of his life, Jack had been medically stable in an unfavorable position. He was a survivor of surgically treated bladder cancer and had a ureteroenterostomy, the bag for which he replaced independently every three days. He also had severe aortic stenosis (obstruction of a heart valve), hypertension, congestive heart failure, chronic lung disease and depression. During the two and a half years before his death, he had been hospitalized three times – all for cardiac problems. However, in the six months before his death, his weight had been stable and he had no chest discomfort. One month before the end, I made a "routine" home visit and was shocked to find that his skinny legs were bloated with fluid and that he seemed to have no energy and was short of breath. His weight was 20 lb heavier than the previous month. Although always fastidious in his appearance, he was now unshaven and unkempt. When I asked him to go to the hospital, he vehemently refused, insisting that he wanted to die in his own home. (I have always been fascinated by the uncanny but usually accurate assurance of patients who may even appear on the mend, let alone deathly ill, to predict their imminent death).

In his presence, I called his daughter who lived in the next town and explained her dad's condition. I told her that he would need massive diuresis and that the resultant urine volume would overwhelm the small capacity of his stomal appliance. His blindness meant that he would require her help to keep him dry and comfortable, and it would be advisable for her to spend at least part of the next few weeks with him in his house. She countered, saying that she was busy now and couldn't come on that day or any other day. She asked me to call her siblings for help with their father. I next called the physician son, only to find that he was halfway around the world on a trip. Calls to another son in Philadelphia were never answered. I finally decided to assume responsibility for care of Jack. I phoned a nursing service to request round-the-clock care to monitor his vital signs and general condition and to empty and change his urinary collection bag. Fortunately, the physician son called the nursing service from 12,000 miles away and assumed financial responsibility for the nursing care. I ordered the appropriate diuretics and visited Jack every other day initially, and then no less than twice per week. The laboratory also visited him at my request twice per week. During that final month, his weight returned to its previously stable value and his shortness of breath decreased so that he was able to move around the first floor of his home with a walker. He continued to affirm that "I don't want to die, but if I do, I want it to be right here with you taking care of me." Throughout these last weeks, none of his five children visited or called either him or me. His 24/7 caretaker called me one day to say that Jack had died suddenly, quietly, comfortably and alone.

Every day I asked myself whether I had done the right thing by expending so much in the way of effort and medical resources on a patient whose death was already imminent and whose family had at best neglected and at worst abandoned him. So far, I have concluded that I acted correctly and that I could not have acted otherwise. My special relationship with Jack, his expressed desire to have me take care of him, and the apparent dissolution of his family ties at the end mandated my intervention. The fact that his children never stopped me from doing so makes me feel that they were glad that I was doing the job that they could not or would not do. But did I go too far in briefly extending the life of a person who was dying and for whom there was no hope of rescue? I can only answer that Jack told me on many occasions that he wanted to live. As his physician, it was my responsibility to make his remaining life as comfortable as possible, and I have no doubt that I accomplished this. Jack was not demented. As long as his decision-making capacity was unimpaired, wouldn't he have had the "fundamental right of self-determination in matters affecting one's own person" of English common law? The answer is *yes*! Too often, decisions about dying patients' welfare are made by physicians and family members acting in concert without input from the patient. Jack died in full command of his admittedly limited destiny.

Moral dilemmas arise in so many different forms. Gary and his devoted family forced me to make an ethical decision that I had not invited and which I did not take any pleasure in making. Gary is an 18-year-old boy who was in a motor vehicle accident one year prior to my visit and suffered a traumatic brain injury that left him with the mentality of a three-month-old baby. Gary's mother had cared for him superbly, and as a result he had not developed pressure ulcers, pneumonia, joint contractures or any of the other complications to which bed-bound patients are prone. Gary did not respond to auditory stimuli, but his mom ardently believed that not only did he respond but also he turned his head in response to his name. Neither I nor any member of the family had ever been able to verify this behavior, but the mother was always so upbeat and her belief in her son's improvement was so strong that no one dared to contradict her.

Gary's mother took advantage of a ruling by the Philadelphia Board of Education that allowed him to obtain daily verbal instruction (or as she put it, "verbal stimulation") until he was 21 years old. I saw those instructors sit in the family's kitchen drinking coffee and telling jokes and stories. When the Board of Education, at the mother's request, asked me to approve another year of "instruction" for Gary, I declined. The nurse at the Board told me that she agreed with me and applauded my decision, but that her hands were administratively tied. When I spoke to the mother about my decision, she discharged me and procured another doctor.

Philadelphia's ruling, in this instance, makes no distinction between those who can benefit from home instruction and those who can't. Even Gary's egregious example would not move anyone to question ways of making the ruling more responsive to individual circumstances. Although money saved from such poorly planned expenditures could be put to better use with better outcomes, the administrative cost of altering this statute and the cost of defense against suits by individuals and special interest groups who feel that they have not been treated fairly would probably far exceed the savings. I can understand Philadelphia's unwillingness to alter this delicate balance, but I nevertheless registered my futile objection to the status quo. Although I would have liked to continue my contact with Gary's family, I did not want to do so when I finally realized that my visits were only appreciated when I was expected to sanction expensive and useless educational therapy.

Sometimes a dilemma is faced by the patient and caregivers rather than by me personally. When the patient's "antagonist" is the federal government or a huge institution, forced submission frequently occurs for the patient and caregivers. Several such events confirmed for me the primacy of business and the "bottom line" in today's patient care. I have almost daily experiences with the powers behind the medical scene (Medicare, HMOs and insurance companies) that frequently dictate how I practice and what care my patients receive. These organizations are monolithic and impersonal. It is usually impossible to reason with them because their decisions are cloaked in a seamless mantle of rules and regulations whose authors are never available for discussion. These decisions are generic and are meant to apply to "every-patient" but not to the individual. It is difficult and often infuriating to attempt to deliver personalized care in an environment that is fettered by unforgiving rules administered by people who are either nameless and faceless or, even when sympathetic to my patients' plights, are not empowered to effect a change or even an exception.

I had taken care of Alice, a 75-year-old woman with a recent stroke that primarily affected her mobility, for the past year. She spent her life either in bed or sitting on the edge of her bed, but could hold interesting conversation. During a routine breast examination, I discovered a mass in her left breast. I sent her to a surgeon who obtained the necessary radiological localization and scheduled her for surgery.

Surgery was scheduled for a Tuesday, with pre-op lab tests to be done the preceding Thursday. The patient's daughter asked the surgeon's office to arrange the pre-op studies to be done at 6.00 a.m. on the day of surgery, so that Alice wouldn't have to be moved from her second-floor bedroom and transported by ambulance on two separate occasions. The surgeon, the patient, her family and I all thought that this was a reasonable request. However, the hospital refused this simple accommodation because Medicare would not reimburse the hospital for pre-op labs performed on the day of surgery.

I just can't figure out whom to blame for this travesty. Is it Medicare for its inability to comprehend that they spend more on two ambulance trips than on one set of lab tests? Or is it the hospital administration for not donating those lab tests to save the patient and her family this inconvenience at a time when their thoughts were preoccupied with the surgery? In either case, fault lies with the attempt to reduce management of all human predicaments to a single protocol. This reduces the overseers of the protocol to mindless and guiltless custodians of the status quo, and deforms the occasional square-peg patient into a round-hole shape.

On another occasion, I was confronted with Maria, an 83-year-old Filipino woman and member of an HMO, who had a symptomatic urinary tract infection for which an antibiotic was indicated. I phoned an order for an antibiotic into the patient's pharmacy, but was called by the patient the next day asking why I had not contacted the pharmacy. When I called the pharmacist, I was told that the HMO had refused the request because the antibiotic was not on their formulary. I then requested another antibiotic. However, Maria called the following day (a Sunday) to find out why she had again not received her antibiotic. When I called the pharmacy, I was told that the HMO had once again refused the drug, this time because the patient had exceeded her drug allowance for the year. The pharmacist said that he would call the HMO the next day to get special permission for Maria to get the antibiotic. I asked him to please supply her with two antibiotic capsules to last her until he could obtain that permission. However, despite the use of logic and eventually pure begging, I was able to obtain only one capsule from the pharmacist. (The HMO gave Maria her full therapeutic supply the next day.)

Who was responsible for this shameful impasse? Was it the pharmacist who had notified neither the patient nor me that two antibiotic requests had been rejected? Or did the fault lie with the HMO for being unavailable on a Sunday to handle Maria's special plight when both the pharmacist and I were on call and eager to help her?

Esther was a 69-year-old woman who had had bone cancer pain for the past year and had received both chemotherapy and radiation to her lumbar spine for intractable cancer pain. At my first visit to her, she was incontinent and required diapers, an indispensable but expensive accessory and one for which she needed to pay out of pocket. However, she also needed fentanyl patches to control her increasing back pain. Because she was covered only by Medicare, her fentanyl was also self-pay.

At that initial visit on a Friday evening, Esther had just run out of both diapers and fentanyl and didn't have enough money to pay for both. She opted for the diapers, realizing the literally painful consequences of that decision.

I left her house on the verge of tears and could barely wait to tell my wife and sons of the human tragedy that I had just witnessed. Is there any justifiable reason why such indignity and an impossible choice should be visited upon anyone?

Finally, the story of Alan and his wife Lynne merits consideration and study. Alan, a 46-year-old man, came under my care five years ago after he fell from a ladder and sustained severe fractures of his pelvis and right leg. He spends most of his time in a wheelchair and is able to hobble only with a rolling walker. He ventures out of his house only to visit an emergency room. Alan also has asthma, for which he needs respiratory "rescue" with inhaled medication several times per week, and hemochromatosis.

Alan had not worked at his job long enough to obtain medical insurance. The total income of the family has been his state-allotted medical assistance of almost $16,000 per year, which goes towards mortgage payments, food, clothes, medications and other very basic necessities. His devoted wife has been his sole caregiver. One year ago she took a menial job to increase their income and to qualify for medical insurance. Although she would rather have worked full-time for benefits, her employer hired her for just less than half-time, but then demanded just $38\frac{1}{2}$ hours' work per week from her, rendering her ineligible for medical benefits.

Two months ago, Lynne tripped and fell in the street, sustaining a fracture of both bones of her lower right leg. She was taken to a Philadelphia hospital that refused to operate on her because she had neither insurance nor savings, and sent her home. She lay in her house for two weeks in severe pain, unable to afford effective pain medication. Her husband gave her two ibuprofen tablets per day from his own slender supply, one on arising and another at bedtime in the hope that she might have a restful night's sleep (she never did). A friend informed her about a free clinic, which sent her to another hospital that performed the necessary surgery. When she applied for state medical assistance, she was told that her husband's meager income disqualified her from receiving assistance. She now gets around on crutches with a long brace on her right leg, but has been unable to afford adequate pain medication. Her husband has recently been *her* caregiver, and cooks and cleans the house to the best of his ability from his wheelchair.

I was unaware of the family's recent plight when I made a routine home visit to Alan a short while ago. Lynne is not my patient, but when she related their story I felt a combination of anguish and anger, the latter at my profession in general and at my colleagues in particular for acquiescing in this inhumanity. I had felt similarly towards Nazi soldiers who had killed innocent people and then claimed that they were only following orders.

Our office employs a social worker three days per week at our own expense. Although Lynne is not my patient, I could not allow her and her husband to founder without support. Our social worker connected them with a charitable agency that delivers meals, another agency that furnishes volunteers to do household chores, a group that supplies generic medications to the poor at affordable prices, and a state legal agency that will work with the hospital to help pay her bills. Throughout this odyssey, Lynne maintained a brave and cheerful attitude. When I expressed how ashamed I was of my profession, she smiled and said "It's not your fault, Doc. It's the system." No one could have expressed it better.

The Patient With an Unsuspected Rich Past

Old patients are usually the most interesting members of society. They have had the most experiences, recount and embellish them in the most fascinating terms, and often have photographs or household decorations that tell their history even when they are no longer able to speak for themselves.

At the risk of being labeled as sexist, I feel that there is an almost universal desire for women to flirt. Flirtation keeps women feeling feminine and young, and this need never disappears, no matter how old the woman. Most of my patients have told me from time to time how well I look. I often reply with "And you are a flirt." The ladies usually react like young coquettes, turning away with shy smiles and looking towards the floor. And then I follow up with "My wife is very jealous and when I tell her about you, she's says she's going to come here and whip your butt." This immediately produces gales of laughter. One of my octogenarians laughingly told me to "watch out for those chippies on the street." These elderly women never seem to lose their interest in men or in male–female repartee. In line with this, I have yet to step into the bathroom of even my oldest patients without finding a bottle of cologne or some other feminine fragrance. If it is not in the bathroom, the spray bottle will be on their night table.

Many times I have also talked to elderly women who are either widowed, divorced or single about their possible interest in a serious binding relationship with a man. They usually give pat, well-worn answers such as "No, I've had my share of that" or "Only if he's rich." Sometimes, especially when I have asked that question of a group of women, feminine group psychology seems to take over as they answer "We don't want those old men. We ladies go out to lunch and they sit sleeping and drooling in their chairs." We've all seen similar disdainful group reactions directed at the male sex from gaggles of grade school girls, secondary school sirens or mature mademoiselles or matrons. Closing my eyes, I can imagine these same lively dowagers as flirtatious teenagers engaging in the "eternal battle of the sexes." *Cherchez la femme.*

Sometimes, because of or even in response to these verbal interchanges, I am challenged to try my own hand in the "eternal battle." A short while ago, I went to an assisted living facility to keep a routine appointment. My patient, slightly balmy but oh so delightful, descended the staircase in a gypsy-like outfit complete with a colorful, flowing skirt, a flowered kerchief around her head, rings on many fingers and varied lengths of bead strings hanging from her wrinkled neck. I told her how beautiful she looked and she replied with the expected "Thank you." At this point, divinely inspired, I said "Does the sun need to thank an admirer who appreciates its splendor?" There was silence and then an audible simultaneous gasp from all my patient's friends in the waiting room, and the ear-splitting grin on her face made my day.

Likewise, the unexpected depth of knowledge, wisdom or accomplishment of patients who show no external hint of such hidden gems sometimes floors me. When visiting my patients, I often remember Thomas Gray's "Elegy" and a "flower ... born to blush unseen."

I couldn't wait to get home to write about Elizabeth. I had taken care of her for one and a half years, but had not really got to know her until recently. Elizabeth is 80 years old and has hypertension, atrial fibrillation, insulin-dependent diabetes mellitus and a history of stroke. Joint contractures resulting from the latter have limited her world to either a bed or a gerichair. She is mentally intact and a brilliant conversationalist. Her sister is her caregiver and constant companion. Neither of them has ever married, and each is the other's only relative.

One day, Elizabeth, without prompting from either her sister or me, decided to show me a book of old photographs. She had joined the Waves in 1943 and subsequently had a 20-year career in the Navy, during which she rose to the rank of CPO (chief petty officer) storekeeper, the top rank for enlisted personnel. The photographs showed her to have been tall (she topped the women surrounding her and was as tall as many of her male companions), blonde and very beautiful. Moreover, she was a champion golfer at a time when women were not noted for athletic achievement, and she led her Wave golf team to victory over their other service counterparts. I saw 50-year-old photos of Elizabeth on the links playing with captains and even admirals. One would never connect the vision in those old photos with the thin, shriveled woman with scissored legs in her gerichair, were it not for her sparkling talk, her engaging sense of humor and a definite trace of authority in her voice.

Rose is a 93-year-old Afro-American woman with hypertension and end-stage renal disease. She was telling me how miserable she felt because she no longer had the physical capability to do things she had routinely done a few short years ago. Now I love poetry, and I adore quoting geriatric-oriented poems to receptive patients when the occasion arises. Sensing an opportune moment, I recited the first stanza of Robert Browning's "Rabbi ben Ezra" ("Grow old along with me ...") without mentioning the author's name. Can you imagine my astonishment when Rose responded by saying "That's beautiful, and I also love Elizabeth Barrett Browning's poems"?

This incident underscored a couple of lessons that I often tell my house staff but which I had temporarily forgotten. First, never pigeonhole anyone into a stereotype. Secondly, remember that the most abject person facing you may have had an unexpectedly rich past, and all of them have rich histories to tell.

This is a good opportunity to recall several incidents from my home visit practice in Philadelphia that only serve to emphasize the error of reducing populations to stereotypes. I had finished my last home visit in North Philadelphia on a cold, snowy February evening at 7.30 p.m., and came out to find that, although I could start my parked car, I could not move it off a patch of ice and snow. I tried to roll the car back and forth, to no avail. The engine noise carried throughout the neighborhood. I was alone and nobody was on the street. Suddenly, as if on cue, five doors opened and several young men emerged, each carrying a shovel. They introduced themselves and then started to place cardboard under the wheels and dig my car out. I asked for one of their shovels and we all joined in. After 15 minutes, we extricated the car. I thanked them all and truly felt that they were as happy as I was that my car had been freed.

On another occasion, I had accidentally left my car trunk open before visiting a patient. When I emerged from the house, a neighborhood resident whom I had never met before was standing by my car. He explained that he was watching the car lest anyone should take anything. I thanked him, and that thanks was the only payment he would accept.

I can cite many instances when, while driving or walking through unfamiliar neighborhoods, I have asked some rough-looking young men the location of a house or street. These young men have often taken me to my destination rather than merely describing its location.

When I have recounted these events to medical colleagues or to other acquaintances, I'm often met with mournful clucks as they say "Too bad you have to work in those areas." No explanation suffices to convince them that working in "those areas" is a rewarding experience both medically and socially. Home visit nurses, physical therapists and their home visit colleagues need no convincing. They have had similar experiences, and each of them has their own rich stories to tell.

Arthur was a 75-year-old man with spina bifida. At the time when I became his physician, he had no family, as his parents and siblings had died and he had never married. He lived in a subsidized apartment house for seniors. His parents had always encouraged him to perform to the limits of his capability. When he was a child, two boys hired by his parents ferried him to and from school daily in a cart. Eventually he was fitted with braces and learned to walk with two canes. He graduated from high school and then worked in a plant, rising to the rank of foreman. Arthur was respected by everyone who knew him. He always spoke quietly, without bitterness or envy, but with underlying experience, authority and, when appropriate, a good sense of humor. Unfailingly good-natured, he assisted his less capable neighbors with their income tax preparations.

Six months before he died, Arthur began to cough up blood. I obtained a portable chest X-ray in his apartment that revealed a large centrally placed left lung mass. A guided needle biopsy confirmed cancer, and he underwent a course of radiation therapy. His bloody cough stopped permanently and, although he continued to dwindle, he was never again troubled by either pain or shortness of breath. Arthur died in his apartment and was cared for by his neighbors to the end.

Walter is a delightful 85-year-old man with an air of respectful impudence. Although never formally educated, he is learned, well read and has a great sense of wit and humor. He is also a retired railroad worker and a devotee of fine scotch whiskey. He had been largely house bound due to a combination of alcohol abuse, chronic lung disease and osteoarthritis, but sent a friend to the store for Johnny Walker (Black Label only) and to the library for books. I have found him reading Oliver Goldsmith, Emily

Dickinson and Robert Louis Stevenson. He had recently completed *Kidnapped* and *The Master of Ballantrae*. I suggested that he should read Stevenson's *A Child's Garden of Verses*, too, and on my next visit he told me how much he had enjoyed that.

After years of trying to convince Walter to go and live with his daughter (who wanted this) and after many hospital admissions for falls and lung disease exacerbations, he puckishly consented to take a neuropsychiatric examination with the understanding that should he prove to be mentally incompetent, he would live with his daughter, but should he be declared competent, he would continue to live alone. I had little hope that he would flunk this test. His MMSE (Mini Mental State Examination – a rudimentary test for dementia) score was 30/30 (perfect). Of course, he passed the more difficult and discerning neuropsychiatric examination with flying colors. Nevertheless, after he had been discharged from hospital, he finally consented to live with his daughter's family in New Jersey. She doesn't allow him to drink officially, but I feel confident that his charm keeps a generous flow of Johnny Walker burbling his way.

I saw Emily, an 83-year-old woman with hypertension, peripheral vascular disease and severe dementia (she didn't know the year, her own birthday or the address at which she had lived for more than 50 years), just once. She lay in bed fondling a large stuffed teddy bear and "conversing" with it. On her night table lay the inevitable bottles of toilet water – Chanel #5 and Poison. After obtaining a basic medical history from her son and examining her, I asked her, without really expecting a reasonable reply, where she had worked. Her persona changed as she answered in a firm, cultured voice, "I was a supervisor at the Philadelphia DPA." Then, realizing that I might not know those initials, she said, "Department of Public Affairs ... and I had a large staff under me." Following that glimmer of authority in her old, accustomed tone of voice, she returned to her teddy bear. Her son, who had previously confirmed his mother's important administrative position, called five days later to tell me that his mother had just died. I will never forget my few minutes with that marvelous woman whom I wished I had known in her heyday.

And then there is Sally, a 76-year-old woman with hypertension, insulin-dependent diabetes, congestive heart failure, morbid obesity and severe osteoarthritis, who spends most of her time lying on her bed or sitting in it clothed in exquisite nightgowns. Her voice is always soft and honey smooth, even when conveying displeasure. In her younger days she earned her living as a "madam" in the very house where I now see her. She often regales me with lively escapades from her past, laced with gambling, guns and her special financial relationship with the local police. She has always used tasteful vocabulary when describing her former work.

However, Sally is now genuinely religious. Although she accepts my medical explanations of her conditions and unfailingly takes my prescribed medications, she always affirms prayer and God as the major reasons for her medical stability. I recently told her that she reminded me of Mary Magdalene. She immediately laughed uproariously in the manner of her former lifestyle and agreed with me, simultaneously musing that she was not sorry for a single day of her former life. On my departure, she looked at me seriously and said "You really care."

My Relationship to Patients with Diabetes Mellitus

I have had insulin-dependent diabetes mellitus for the past 38 years. Throughout my career I have taken care of many diabetic patients. I enjoy talking to them, giving them advice and taking joy in their happiness when their clinical situation improves. Likewise, I know that they trust me. They have never had to explain to me what hypoglycemia feels like. When I tell them to carry tubes of cake icing to forestall such episodes, I love to see their faces light up with that "Eureka!" look. They realize that my advice is tempered by 38 years of trial-and-error experience, and they also know that I have a successful career and family and that I have not had any diabetic complications. I know that I've been a role model for many of my diabetic patients throughout my career and, as I approach my sixty-eighth birthday, these patients still relate to me in a very personal way. Two of my diabetic patients have had a special impact on me.

Jim is a 71-year-old man with the unenviable chronic disease load of insulin-dependent diabetes, hypertension, stroke with right-sided paralysis (but with cognitive and speech preservation), arteriosclerotic heart disease, congestive heart failure, severe peripheral arterial disease and urge urinary incontinence. He is a retired policeman and his son is also a policeman. Jim lives with his charming wife, whose financial acumen has enabled them to purchase several rental properties. His wife, who was not my patient, was found to have a large kidney mass (which proved benign at surgery). Prior to her surgery, I had arranged for Jim's care while she would be convalescing. I had brought Jim's diabetes under control to the point where his measured blood sugars were largely within normal limits. His blood pressure and congestive heart failure are now under good control. I also obtained a device for him that prevented foot drop and allowed him to walk safely. Having accomplished that, I started him on medications that enabled him to walk pain-free for several blocks without fear of losing his urine while walking.

After these events, which had occurred over a period of several years, Jim, his wife and I were talking after I had completed an examination, when Jim turned to me and said "Dr. Stillman, I feel like we're almost married." My only response was to hug him, and that hug was heartily returned. The three of us then laughed and hugged each other. What a wonderful feeling to have been accepted as a part of their innermost family!

Paul was a 57-year-old insurance executive and body builder who had lost 130 lb during the past year due to an abdominal malignancy which had spread to his spine and lungs. His major problem was unremitting severe bone pain, which radiotherapy and powerful pain medications had failed to relieve. When I first became his physician, Paul had just two weeks to live. At my initial visit, he was able to talk to me only with great effort, due to pain. He kept his fists clenched and his eyelids shut, but did his best to answer my questions.

However, Paul also had insulin-dependent diabetes, although for the two weeks before his death he had not taken insulin because of his weight loss and reduced intake. During our first meeting, I informed him (as I always have done when I meet new diabetic patients) that I, too, had diabetes. Shortly after the start of the interview, I became hypoglycemic with fuzzy thought and loss of concentration. Although his eyes were closed and he was in terrible pain, he told me to go into his kitchen and drink some orange juice which I would find in his refrigerator. I followed his advice, came back to him and thanked him. He smiled, the only time I ever saw him do so. Two weeks later he had died, his pain relieved by huge doses of morphine.

Hospice and the Dying Patient

My practice has a rapid turnover, usually because my patients die. Many of my patients and their families have never heard of hospice. They may think it's a play on the word "hospital." Even when they have heard of the word, they often don't understand the concept of hospice and what it tries to do. Hospice is truly one of the best-kept secrets in the United States. When I explain to a terminally ill patient and caregiver that hospice offers a "good death", and explain that this is a goal that not all people realize, their interest is perked. When I go on to explain that hospice is a combination of physicians, nurses, psychologists, social workers and religious people working together to achieve that goal, and that their contact with and support of the patient's family continues after the patient dies, their interest is further stimulated. I then go on to say that everyone is entitled to hospice benefits for at least six months through Social Security benefits. These benefits include free medications and durable medical equipment (e.g. hospital beds, commodes, air mattresses, etc.) and home health aides at least three times per week. In the United States, hospice care is almost always administered in the patient's home. In a few instances, some hospices maintain free-standing facilities where dying patients can be taken for care in their last days. (Free-standing hospices are characteristic of hospice care in the United Kingdom.) The families, including the patients, are relieved to know that many hospices also offer respite care where the patient can be cared for in a skilled nursing facility for up to five days per month to allow the caregiver free time. Finally, I tell the patient and their family that even if a patient survives for longer than six months, I have rarely seen hospices discontinue their program and benefits for any patient. By this time, consent is virtually assured. However, I have noted that some ethnic groups (e.g. Asian-Americans) have been slow to accept hospice, preferring to shoulder the responsibility of terminal care for their loved ones alone or in concert with other family members.

I think I can now relate the stories of four patients for whom hospice meant a great deal, but in very different ways.

Zora was a 67-year-old Afro-American woman who was morbidly obese to the extent that she was bed-bound and able to sit on the side of the bed only with great effort and if assisted by several family members. She also had insulin-dependent diabetes mellitus and hypertension, and had undergone left mastectomy for cancer three years prior to her death. She had no evidence of metastasis at the time of surgery and, because of her obesity, had not been able to return for regular oncological visits. She was fully aware of her surroundings and was able to converse quite well. Six months before her death, Zora, while sitting on the side of the bed, had fallen to the floor, and had experienced severe left hip pain as a result. I arranged for ambulance transport for hip and chest films as well as a nuclear medicine bone scan which demonstrated multiple metastatic lesions in the ribs, pelvis, femur, humeri, scapulae and skull. Zora had suffered a pathological fracture. The ensuing admission and oncological consultation resulted in the addition of hormonal medication, which Zora's daughters gave to her at home.

Zora's three daughters were very devoted to her. All three were Muslim and wore full-length black gowns that revealed only their hands and eyes. After I had controlled Zora's pain, I introduced the hospice concept to her and her daughters (each of whom took turns to stay with her 24 hours per day). Although Zora regarded the idea favorably, only one of her daughters shared her opinion, while the other two, hoping that their mom would be a long-term survivor, resisted hospice. As the weeks wore on, and despite faithful delivery of anti-breast cancer hormonal therapy, Zora's multiple metastatic sites began to hurt, necessitating an increase in pain medication. Moreover, new areas of bony pain occurred that had not been recognized on the bone scan. Zora's appetite also began to fail. The two daughters who had resisted hospice now called me to make the appropriate arrangements.

When hospice arrived, the nurses moved Zora's bed from an interior room of the house to a window on the first floor so that she could enjoy daylight and watch activity on the street. Their personnel built a strong relationship with Zora and her daughters. The hospice nurse visited their home three times per week and called me frequently for directions for diabetes and pain control. I continued to visit Zora every two to three weeks and was in frequent telephone contact with her family. Eventually she became progressively more sleepy and then passed away without pain. A few weeks after Zora's death, each of her daughters called me to express gratitude for my advice and patience in bringing them to a decision in favor of hospice.

Incidentally, I have never encountered any family or caregiver who was dissatisfied with hospice services.

Sarah was a 62-year-old Jewish woman with breast cancer who had been treated four years previously with mastectomy and eventual hormonal therapy, chemotherapy and radiation therapy for liver and painful bone metastases. Her bone metastases had actually increased in size despite continued therapy. She and her devoted husband were poor and lived alone with their cat in an apartment on the third floor of a walk-up building. They had never had children. Their only relative was Sarah's sister, who lived in Philadelphia and with whom they were in frequent telephone contact. Sarah never went out of her apartment except to be taken to her oncologist by ambulance.

Over a period of a few weeks, Sarah developed a stumbling gait and headaches that were unrelieved by acetaminophen. Her oncologist obtained a brain MRI scan that revealed multiple brain metastases, and then suggested that she should receive further hormonal therapy. I talked to the oncologist and indicated that this might be an opportune time to consider hospice. The oncologist refused to consider that option until Sarah had received the "full benefit of hormonal therapy." I met with Sarah and her husband in their home, discussed Sarah's prognosis with them, outlined the possible therapeutic courses (including hospice) and their potential benefits and drawbacks, and was gratified when they opted for hospice. Incidentally, hospice should not be regarded as an option only when there are no further therapeutic options. It is a reasonable choice when other so-called options have virtually no chance of affecting the patient's course and would only prolong their discomfort or pain without offering a chance of recovery or even palliation.

Sarah died at home peacefully with her husband by her side. She had been pain-free since hospice arrived two months before her death. When she died, hospice and I had anticipated that her husband, the more retiring member of the couple, might need assistance in adjusting to his wife's death. This assistance was indeed required within 24 hours, and hospice was there immediately to obtain help from the Jewish Family Service.

Jane was a 76-year-old woman with terminal emphysema who had been married for more than 50 years. She had been a Democratic committeewoman in Philadelphia for 30 years, and her poverty-stricken home's walls were festooned with tributes from familiar past and present local political names. The couple had lived in their house for the past 41 years. The "neighborhood had changed", and a significant number of drug suppliers and their clientele now lived close by. However, the local citizenry, in acknowledgement of Jane's contributions to neighborhood welfare (funding school libraries, cleaning the streets, etc.), were solicitous about her and were friendly with the couple.

Jane's 83-year-old husband and primary (indeed sole) caregiver was a veteran of the Battle of the Bulge in World War Two. After the war, he enrolled in the military police and married Jane in 1948. After retiring from the military, he worked as a guard for a local industry, and had retired 20 years before. The couple had one daughter who had married and moved to Ohio. They had several grandchildren whom they had never seen. They also hadn't seen their daughter for four years, since she returned to Philadelphia only to attend her mother-in-law's funeral.

Jane was already on hospice when I arrived to take over as her physician. She was too short of breath to either eat or talk, but she clearly understood everything that was said to her. Her husband privately told me that he had been urged by friends and other health care workers to place his wife in a nursing home because they felt that he was not up to caring for her. He had refused to do so. With tears in his eyes, he told me how much he loved her and how wonderful she had always been to him. He realized that she had no more than a few days, perhaps two weeks at most, to live. He was bent over when walking, but he would sleep on a sofa by the side of her hospital bed at home, sit near her, talk to her and take care of her. A nursing home for her would mean new surroundings and new faces, which would frighten her. Moreover, he had sold his car years ago, so would not be able to drive to see her daily. No, he said, he would never place her in a nursing home.

Hospice made a great difference to Jane's comfort during her final days. The nurse instructed her husband about administration of morphine to sedate her should she become anxious or frightened while severely short of breath. She also explained to him ways to control her diarrhea. A home health aide came in daily to bathe her, tidy the small home and prepare food for

Jane's husband. Jane died peacefully with her life's companion holding her in his arms.

Edward was a 67-year-old Afro-American man who had hypertension, insulin-dependent diabetes mellitus and a stroke from which he had made a reasonably good recovery. His speech was unimpaired, but he still had difficulty dragging his right leg up and down stairs. Because of this, he stayed mostly by himself in a crowded second-floor bedroom of his house, coming down only to eat. He lived in the house with his wife, his son and several grandchildren. He had a long history of smoking cigarettes and had had a persistent cough for years.

After I had been Edward's physician for two years, he told me that he had recently coughed up blood. I sent him to a hospital for a chest X-ray, which disclosed a huge lung mass. The radiologist told me that his number one, two and three diagnoses were lung cancer, and that his other diagnostic choices were immaterial. I went to Edward's home to explain the gravity and prognosis of the situation, and his wife, whom I scarcely knew after two years, said to him "You know what that means? It means you gonna die!" I was struck by the unexpected vehemence of that statement and the fury of the person who delivered it. Edward later told me that his wife, son and grandchildren ignored him and that it was his wife who had turned them all against him. He never acknowledged any blame for the relationships between himself and his family. I asked him whether he had any other family members or friends whom he might like me to call to visit him. He said that he had no friends, but told me about his minister brother in Wilmington, Delware, whom he would like to see. When I called this brother, he was polite but told me that he had tried to see Edward for years, but that Edward had not accepted his visits or invitations. Nevertheless, he said he would try to drive up to see him – but never did.

Edward accepted hospice gratefully. He lost his appetite and rapidly lost 40 lb. However, his cough was controlled, he never became short of breath and he remained pain-free. He became increasingly morose and bitter. He changed his will and directed that his meager estate be left to charity. He moved out of his house to a free-standing hospice where he died, visited only by his hospice nurse and myself.

Ethnic Vignettes

One of the most "fun" parts of my job is my daily contact with so many different cultures and, not infrequently, the surprising intermingling of those cultures in a single individual. I have already mentioned several of my contacts with culturally diverse people, but want to present here some of my most memorable experiences in this area.

When I was eight years old, my parents sent me to school after my regular day school classes to learn Yiddish. I was fluent in Yiddish by age ten but, with virtually no opportunity to use the language, my fluency declined dramatically during my teens. However, when I became a home visit geriatrician, I discovered pockets of patients scattered throughout Philadelphia whose primary language, despite years in this country, was still Yiddish. I bought an English–Yiddish dictionary (not easy to come by) and began to browse through and refer to it after I had seen elderly Jewish patients whose history I had not completely comprehended. Eventually my Yiddish fluency returned and I now sometimes surprise myself with spontaneous recourse to vocabulary that I have not used in more than 50 years.

On my journey to that point, I spoke Yiddish haltingly with interspersed German words (relics of my college days). However, my massacre of Yiddish didn't stop an elderly Jewish patient who did not speak English from bursting into tears (of joy) when I spoke to her. Conversely, another elderly Jewish woman who spoke Yiddish and English fluently laughed good-naturedly at my atrocious Yiddish grammatical errors. I treasure equally the vivid memories of Jewish patients who kiss my ring, elderly Hispanic patients who kiss my hands or press their face against my hand, elderly black patients who pray for me, or the Filipino caregiver of her elderly mom who invited me to her daughter's wedding.

In my younger, inexperienced days of medical practice, I had looked askance at the concept of faith healing. Of course, I now realize that much of what I accomplish is faith healing. Most of my patients not only have a strong faith in God but also in me as an agent of the divine will. I don't regard myself as such an agent, but it is nevertheless difficult to live up to these expectations.

Grace is a 92-year-old woman from a strict Irish Catholic background who lives alone and is adoringly and frequently visited by her many grand- and great-grandchildren. Although she has hypertension, mild deafness and borderline dementia, she remains one of my healthier patients. At my very first visit, Grace had told me of numbness in her right hand that appeared immediately after arising, lasted for about 30 minutes and then disappeared until the next morning. She had no neck pain or similar symptoms in her other limbs, and the sensation was not accompanied by weakness. Physical examination, invariably conducted in the late afternoon, was always normal. I suspected that Grace's complaint might have something to do with the position in which she slept, but could not prove it. I also didn't feel that any medication would be either advisable or helpful for a sensation that was so brief and which did not produce disability.

And then came a revelation! Grace pulled forth a mini-bottle of a clear liquid for which she had sent to France and for which she had paid only five dollars. It was "holy water from Lourdes." Grace rubbed a few drops from that bottle on to her right hand each morning and her numbness disappeared immediately. I could never have done better at so little cost and without any side-effects. I've often wondered how many of the medications and how much of the advice that I dispense act in a similar manner to "holy water."

A few years ago I met Eula, my first Afro-American Native American. She was a card-carrying member of the Nanicoke–Lenape tribe, and her grandmother had been a full-blooded Native American. Eula had attended tribal meetings as a young girl. She said that there was a significant population of Afro-American Native Americans in Philadelphia. I subsequently confirmed this and now have two additional Afro-American Native American patients.

Eula was a 79-year-old woman who 50 years previously had been found to have a hemangioma located in her left thigh and buttock. The tumor was apparently too massive to remove surgically or reduce with radiation even when it was initially found. It gradually grew and invaded her spinal column and left leg, causing severe pain. She underwent surgery at age 36 years to relieve the pressure on the spinal cord. The tumor bulk was not significantly reduced but, in the surgical aftermath, Eula suffered paraplegia at the level of the tenth thoracic vertebra, and incontinence of both bowel and bladder. She also experienced neurogenic pain that was only partially relieved with large doses of opiates, which she was unable to afford. When I first took on her care, I sent her again to a vascular surgeon and radiotherapist, adding an interventional radiologist and laser specialist to the bevy of subspecialist physicians she had seen. All of them reported that the tumor was too massive and located in too dangerous and sensitive an area for them to even contemplate reducing the tumor mass, let alone afford pain relief. In addition, Eula had fallen out of her wheelchair at age 61 years, and as a result required surgical repair of a hip fracture. Finally, she was an inveterate smoker and suffered from chronic lung disease and recurrent pulmonary infections.

Eula spent her waking hours in a wheelchair into and out of which she was able to transfer unaided. On many occasions I witnessed those transfers as she lifted her ponderous left leg with a towel, the two ends of which she grasped in her hands. She had a bladder catheter and relied on stool softeners and herbal laxatives for defecation. She ate and dressed independently, but needed an aide to bathe her and cook for her. A friend did her laundry and shopping. During the two and a half years that I was her physician, Eula developed progressive shortness of breath, even at rest, and later in her course an enlarging, infected and deep sacral pressure ulcer that didn't heal despite intensive attention from wound care nurses, surgical debridement at a hospital, and use of an air mattress. Although Eula was fiercely independent and had always preferred to do as much for herself as possible, she finally and tearfully told me that she could no longer take care of herself, and asked to be sent to a nursing home. I had never expected to hear such a request from her, but within one month I was able to admit her.

After Eula had moved to her nursing home, although I was no longer her physician I maintained contact with her. She survived for four more years in that nursing home. Her pain remained under reasonable control with morphine, and her primary problems proved to be recurrent lung infections and increasing dyspnea. When she no longer had concerns about being alone, buying her medications, cooking her meals, or getting into and out of bed or on to a toilet, she blossomed, mingled with all the other residents, participated in all of the activities, and was visited by her numerous and loving family members. She finally died after a six-week period during which she had shortness of breath from which she could not be extricated. At the end, she refused all further assistance and died peacefully in full possession of all her considerable mental faculties.

In the interim, Eula had taught me much about stoicism in the face of great pain, and about the potential benefit of a nursing home environment. Throughout this book I have noted that in many cases in my experience, nursing home residence is not a reasonable option for the elderly because it is expensive and often seems to be more of an expediency for family members of patients with limited cognitive ability who are unable to care for themselves. Eula's case appears to me to be a happy exception in which a caring and medically sound nursing home environment contributed to an end of life that was vastly improved compared with her years of living independently. Of course, Eula had investigated and chosen nursing home life independently and had not been deposited there by an exhausted caregiver or family. I'm sure that Eula's nursing home experience can be replicated, but only when both the home and the patient are carefully evaluated to ensure that each fully meets the other's needs.

Speaking of ethnic surprises, one of my patients, Joe, is a 96-year-old Afro-American veteran of World War Two who lives in a subsidized black apartment building. When I first came to his apartment, I saw a mezuzah next to the entrance. I was even more surprised when I saw the large number of Hebrew books on his shelves. I couldn't resist the temptation to immediately question him. I had known that black (Falasha) Jews exist, but they came from Ethiopia and this man was American-born.

Joe told me that when the war ended, he sought new meaning in life and, after searching for that meaning, decided to convert to Judaism. His father was a Baptist minister, and although his family turned their backs on him he persisted in learning about Judaism and the Hebrew language. He was circumcised and he speaks, reads and writes Hebrew fluently. He observes all the Jewish holidays and holy days. He certainly knows more about traditional Judaism than I do. He attends a black synagogue and his fellow congregants call him "rabbi", although he has never had formal rabbinical instruction, as a mark of respect for his learning. Joe told me that there is a large black Jewish community in Philadelphia. Subsequently I have met other black Jews who confirm his statement. Joe and I always wish each other "happy holiday" at the time of a Jewish holiday.

Incidentally, 96-year-old Joe has been fluent in conversational Hebrew for decades. He continues to take courses in Hebrew studies at Temple University, and was recently asked by the foreign languages department to instruct an undergraduate section in Hebrew. He replied that he would be delighted to do so but that he first wanted to "take a few more semesters of advanced Hebrew before tackling the teaching assignment." He did so, and is now a member of the Temple University faculty. He also attends several Judaica meetings throughout the year in various parts of the United States, and teaches a Hebrew language seminar two evenings per week across the Delaware River in Camden, New Jersey. To do this, he recrosses the river at night and then both walks and takes public transportation to his apartment house.

Lest anyone think that Joe is a one-sided Judaic "nerd", they would be wrong! He reads several newspapers per day and subscribes to news magazines. He is well spoken and authoritatively knowledgeable about world, national and local events. During my visits to him, we spend at least 20 minutes discussing current events and his most recent social activities. He is also a "people person", has a large number of friends and belongs to many social and political organizations. He and his family have long since been reconciled with each other, and he regularly attends family conclaves. Joe is ageless.

Another of my patients is Yolanda, an 82-year-old Hispanic woman who has lived in the United States since 1952 but who speaks no English. Her husband of over 50 years, Carlos, also a Hispanic-American, is her primary caregiver. Their son, an only child, lives around the corner and assists his father with Yolanda's care. Their home is small, filthy and inhabited by vermin. However, the walls are decorated with many photographs of the couple in their young years together. In the photographs, Carlos is handsome in an American army uniform and Yolanda is vivacious and beautiful. There is also an old picture of Carlos in uniform embracing his mother. A few replicas of famous paintings hang proudly on those grimy walls.

Yolanda has been unable to hold a conversation for at least four years. She speaks, but her son and husband assured me that what she says makes no sense even to them. She requires help with feeding, is unable to walk or even to stand by herself, and is totally incontinent. Her husband does all of the household tasks, including shopping and cooking, as well as changing his wife's diapers. He is short of breath due to chronic lung disease, but has no relief from his wife's constant needs. Yolanda is often awake at night and yells, depriving him of the sleep he so desperately needs.

When I first met her, Yolanda was disheveled and incredibly filthy. After examining her, I concluded that her only disability was severe dementia. I explained my findings to Carlos and their son. They understood the implications of the problem, and Carlos asked whether help for him to care for his wife was available. I told him about PCA (Philadelphia Corporation for the Aging) and explained that his impoverishment would probably qualify him for a full complement of services. But then, in his broken English, Carlos tearfully said, "I no want her to go to crazy house. I want her here with me."

All day long I felt privileged to be invited into the sanctity of this poor home and to see the depth of this long love affair. Those youngsters in the photos could hardly have imagined their lives at this time. But their love was the saving grace in their lives, and I truly felt that if either of them had had the opportunity to change their life, knowing in advance their present situation, neither would have done so. I have had the opportunity to witness many such love affairs, which end tragically but whose totality is reminiscent of great literature or grand opera. Perhaps these relationships that I have seen are "grand" precisely because their drama and emotions, like those of opera, strike a familiar chord in us all.

Two weeks after seeing Yolanda, I procured long-term nursing care and home health aides for this couple for the indefinite future.

Appreciation (or Non-appreciation) of Homebound Patient Problems by Hospital-based or Ambulatory Physicians

I sometimes find that high-powered consultants (of whom I used to be one) or physicians whose entire professional experience occurs within a hospital's walls forget about the *person* whose ailments they are so diligently pursuing. The most flagrant example of such focused "healing" occurred when I directed Joan, an 82-year-old woman with new-onset severe chest pain to the hospital for evaluation for possible heart attack. She also had hypertension, insulin-dependent diabetes mellitus, congestive heart failure and severe peripheral vascular disease. When I first took over her care, she had already had a left above-knee amputation. About one year thereafter, I made an emergency visit to her home after her family phoned to tell me that her remaining foot was painful and discolored. After one look, I called an ambulance and sent Joan to the nearest hospital, where she had her second above-knee amputation. After that, Joan lived on the first floor of her house and was confined to her bed. Her family took good care of her, but all the responsible members either worked or attended school. Even so, with the help of neighbors, Joan was watched almost 24 hours per day, and was lifted from her bed to a wheelchair about twice per week.

When Joan arrived at the hospital, the main teaching hospital of a prominent Philadelphia medical school, a senior cardiologist took over her care. Three days later, he called me to say that she indeed had angina, but had not suffered a heart attack, and that he was going to perform coronary angiography that day. "But", I said, "why not just treat her medically without the invasive procedure? After all, she is bed-bound and doesn't walk anywhere due to her amputations." There was a prolonged, uncomfortable silence, after which the cardiologist managed to stammer that he had not known she was an amputee. Then he recovered and, with some anger, said more assertively "My resident should have told me that!" Of course he was exposed as either not having personally examined Joan or, if he had, being so heart-directed that he had totally neglected to notice that she had no legs. Joan was discharged home that same day without a procedure but on appropriate anti-anginal medication.

In today's technically oriented health care delivery system, too many physicians have either forgotten or neglected to obtain the most valuable diagnostic tool: the detailed medical history. Reasons for this laxity range from inadequate emphasis on and teaching of the medical history in medical school, to a misplaced total reliance on imaging and laboratory procedures as the "gold standard" for diagnosis, and the pressure on physicians by health care delivery organizations to see as many patients as possible in the shortest time possible.

We home care physicians take pride in obtaining detailed medical histories from our patients. We see few patients per day, but we spend exhaustive time with them getting to know them, and we routinely use that knowledge to manage even complex medical problems in their homes. I sometimes see patients who could have avoided expensive hospitalization, multiple procedures and potentially harmful medications if a proper medical history had been obtained prior to admission.

Barbara is an 82-year-old woman who up until recently had always been healthy. She had never been hospitalized, she lived alone and she drove her car all over the city. She and her sister lived across the street from each other, but both were independent and widows of long standing. Each was the other's best friend. On a scorching July day during a memorable heatwave in our city, Barbara's sister found her disoriented and lying on her bed. Barbara had told her sister two days previously that her air conditioner had failed and that she was awaiting the repairman but he had not arrived. The sister had tried to take care of Barbara alone for several weeks. She was able to speak and walk and was not weak, but she was incontinent and often her speech did not make sense. Eventually, finding Barbara's care too demanding, her sister brought her to a local tertiary care hospital. There she received a mega-neurological evaluation, but no evidence of vascular disease, neoplasm or intracranial bleeding was found. She was also evaluated psychiatrically and received three potent drugs for behavior control, on which she was discharged. After discharge, Barbara slept for most of the day but could be aroused to eat or answer questions.

When I first evaluated Barbara four weeks after her hospital discharge, I felt that she had suffered heat encephalopathy when her air conditioner had stopped working. I found no focal neurological deficits. I gradually withdrew her neuropsychiatric drugs, to which she responded by awakening, becoming more conversational, taking her own bath and helping to dry the dishes. She is still incontinent, but this problem has been ameliorated with medication for both bowel and bladder. She will never drive a car again, but accompanies her sister on shopping trips to the mall and for food, and takes accompanied walks through the neighborhood. How much sooner and more expeditiously might this have occurred had the link between Barbara's rapid change in mental status and the heat wave been established at the tertiary care medical center?

I am always amazed by the trust that my patients and their caregivers place in me. It is one thing to write about how that may have happened, but quite another to contemplate it with the respect that it deserves. That trust is given me because my elderly patients know that their welfare is in my hands and that I will do everything possible to ensure that they will not suffer and that they will be treated with the dignity they deserve. It is a responsibility that I do not take lightly. The following story is an example of how I often act as the guardian of the patient and their caregiver, protecting them against well-meaning but useless, costly and potentially harmful academic suggestions from specialist colleagues who have no appreciation of their history.

Sheila was a 53-year-old woman with severe rheumatoid arthritis and rheumatoid lung disease. She had spent 8 of the last 12 months of her life in hospital with recurrent episodes of shortness of breath and pneumonia. Much of that time had been spent in the intensive-care unit (ICU). Although she retained her ability to think and reason, her quality of life had been poor because of unremitting arthritic pain and progressive shortness of breath. Her exercise tolerance was so low that she was only able to move from her bed to a nearby commode, and even this required assistance. During her last prolonged hospitalization for pulmonary insufficiency, she developed a slow heart rate and fainted. She had not had any prior history of cardiac disease. She was rushed to the ICU unresponsive, and was intubated and ventilated. The staff cardiologist, who did not know her or her family (and who had not contacted me for background information), suggested to her daughter that Sheila should have a transvenous pacemaker. His rationale for the procedure was that "the benefits outweigh the risks." Sheila's daughter immediately called me to apprise me of the situation and to ask my advice. I discussed the pros and cons with her, but then explained to her that the pacemaker would benefit her mother's heart but would certainly not benefit her mother or improve her quality of life. The daughter listened to me and refused the pacemaker. Sheila died peacefully a short while later, and her daughter subsequently called me to thank me for my care.

There is one more story of hospital physicians who admit patients whom they don't really know and then order tests and deliver services that don't benefit and may even harm the patient.

Linda was a 73-year-old woman with multiple sclerosis, malnutrition, multiple deep pressure ulcers, right leg arterial insufficiency, steroid osteopenia, Alzheimer's disease and symptomatic gastroesophageal reflux. I list these entities to emphasize the complexity and irreversibility of most of her problems. I had initiated therapy for her reflux disease with a standard acid-reducing medication, and was pleased that this had made her life more bearable. However, just before and during treatment, I had noticed that her hemoglobin level was gradually falling. When her stool was positive for blood, I decided to transfuse her until the acid-reducing pill had had a full opportunity to work. I had tried to accomplish this through a home infusion service, but couldn't find a company willing to transfuse a first-time recipient. I then sent the patient to the nearest hospital emergency room after first explaining to both the patient and her family *and the emergency room staff* the purpose of this referral.

Unfortunately, Linda was subjected to a four-day admission about which I was never informed and whose discharge summary I never received. The unprofessional behavior which has become all too familiar to me in recent years prompted the following letter to the chief of the medical staff of that hospital. The recipient of that letter never contacted me.

Dear Dr. ....,

I am writing to you, the chief medical officer of ... Hospital, to bring to your attention a set of circumstances that recently occurred at your institution that sounds either flagrantly rude and disrespectful, grossly uncaring, or perhaps both.

I am a geriatrician who specializes in home visit care. However, I am board certified and fellowship trained in internal medicine, gastroenterology and geriatrics. On ..., I referred my home visit patient, Linda ..., to the ... Hospital ER for a blood transfusion. She had a low hemoglobin due to slow GI blood loss with massive iron deficiency. Symptomatically, she also had gastroesophageal reflux and, prior to her transfusion, I had initiated therapy with both oral iron and omeprazole [a suppressant of gastric acid production]. Within 11 days of my initial visit and the start of omeprazole, her pyrosis [heartburn] had completely resolved. I had tried to have the transfusion done at home through ... Infusion Co. but, because this was a first transfusion, they suggested that this should be done at the nearest hospital. The patient only consented after I had assured her that this would be an outpatient procedure.

When Linda arrived at the hospital ER, an ER physician informed me that there was no facility at the hospital for giving an outpatient transfusion, and that she would require admission. We both agreed that this antiquated rule sounded like overkill. I asked the physician to contact whoever he needed to in order to ensure that my patient received just her blood and no other gratuitous services, and he said he would do his best. Imagine my shock when Linda's nursing service called me about one week later to ask for the results of her four-day admission, during which she had undergone colonoscopy and esophago-gastroduodenoscopy. The endoscopist had found the historically obvious peptic esophagitis (which he dutifully but needlessly confirmed by biopsy) as well as two tiny colon polyps and a piece of vegetable matter (all, of course, histologically confirmed), none of which was the cause of her anemia. Most significantly, Linda is 73 years old and has severe, progressive multiple sclerosis as well as joint contractures and four severe pressure ulcers, one of which is Stage IV (bone is exposed in the ulcer bed). In addition, she has early dementia (MMSE 23/30), depression, peripheral vascular disease and steroid osteopenia.

Dr. ..., as a gastroenterologist, geriatrician and humanitarian, it was obvious to me not only what could have been but also what should have been accomplished diagnostically. This patient's quality of life, her home situation, and her other chronic conditions besides anemia dictated a more thoughtful, caring and conservative approach than the "damn the torpedoes" double endoscopy approach that she endured at ... Hospital. Moreover, at the very least, the attending physician (who didn't know her at all and had no feeling for her home situation) should have contacted me. After I found out about the admission, I immediately called Dr. .... His answering service took my message and said that he would receive it on his return to the office at about 2 p.m. He has not yet called me back.

I hope that you don't consider this letter as the railings of an old-fashioned 59-year-old physician against the new ethical order. As you will have noticed, I've barely touched the subject of clinical competence, and have largely confined my remarks to manners, morals, and attention that should be paid by physicians to a patient rather than a lab finding. Thank you for hearing me out. I look forward to hearing from you in the near future.

Sincerely,

I never heard from any of the parties involved. The patient died shortly after this admission. However, in all fairness, motivation for performing seemingly unnecessary procedures may involve the hospital physician's possibly inadequate collection of historical data (often readily available from the PCP), the very real fear of many physicians that they need to cover themselves against possible lawsuits by proving that they did everything possible to achieve a diagnosis (even though "everything possible" may be useless and even harmful to a patient), as well as the obvious acquisition of extra fees for procedures. In addition, many more young subspecialists who perform expensive procedures (e.g. cardiologists, gastroenterologists and radiologists) have been trained in recent years, causing an oversupply in major metropolitan areas. The medical rationale for performing procedures may sometimes be stretched by newly minted "proceduralists."

"Running the Gauntlet" of Hospitalization

When my patients were much younger and during my formative years as a young physician, it was common to hospitalize patients for diagnostic evaluation and even for temporary alleviation of social situations at home, or mental distress. These hospital admissions are no longer tolerated unless the admitting physician has outlined his or her *proposed therapeutic plan* for the patient during hospitalization. Utilization review committees determine whether a patient's condition can pass muster, and they now scrutinize all admissions. These committees have been so successful that our hospitals are now often referred to as "acute care facilities." Our hospitals no longer care for chronically ill patients unless an acute exacerbation of their chronic illness occurs.

However, my patients grew up and spent their middle years in an era of essentially unrestricted hospitalization. They have a reverence for hospitals. Also, because they are so frail and, in many instances, isolated, they fear even insignificant symptoms and look to the hospital as the safest and most reliable place to restore them to their baseline health status. They don't realize that hospitals are no longer safe havens for patients with chronic debilitating disease. Thirty years ago, the resident hospital bacteria were still naïve regarding antibiotics and had not yet become today's fearsome survivors. The hospitals that I knew as a young doctor were staffed by a large number of nurses, aides and young nursing students who were directed and had the time to religiously turn truly bed-bound patients from side to side to prevent pressure ulcers. These same personnel would remove all potentially mobile patients from bed and walk them in the halls daily to preserve their muscle strength and mobility and to mobilize their lung secretions and stagnating blood pools. Today, many patients are consigned to bed rest even though they are functionally capable of spending many hours in a chair or even walking. As we know, the dangers of continued bed rest are notorious and include:

1 promotion of pressure ulcers (which may arise in fewer than six hours, but may take many months to heal)
2 loss of muscle strength (deconditioning), which further promotes bed rest

3 stagnation of blood and secretions, leading to lower extremity blood clots (and possibly pulmonary emboli) and pneumonia, respectively
4 dissolution of bones due to disuse, with resultant bony fractures and calcium-containing kidney stones.

The reasons for this de-emphasis on preventive care for the hospitalized elderly are a combination of:

- a severe shortage of nurses due to the short-sighted closure of many nursing schools and the disillusionment of nurses with their working environment leading many to enter a different field
- economic pressures on hospitals which often don't replace retiring or resigning nurses, but instead require the remaining nurses to work harder.

In short, today's infirm elderly do not understand that, for them, hospitals are not as safe as they may have supposed. I have known patients who were ambulatory before hospital admission and who emerged never to walk again, due to deconditioning. Others who had never had a pressure ulcer prior to admission were discharged with multiple deep pressure ulcers. Therapy for these sores often requires further bed rest (to keep the sores free of pressure from the seat of a chair), which leads to increased deconditioning. In addition, placement of a Foley catheter is often necessary to keep these sores dry, and the urinary catheter promotes bladder or kidney infections, often with antibiotic-resistant hospital bacteria. Educating today's elderly homebound about the need to avoid hospitalization unless absolutely necessary – and even then only for treatment of a *serious acute disease* – may be difficult. I feel that this re-education should be the individual physician's responsibility and not that of the government or the media.

"The Ties That Bind"

We all know stories of how people who live together for a long time become so close that they think of and say things simultaneously, and may even begin to look alike. Their thought processes and value systems may become indistinguishable from each other's. It seems that this becomes increasingly obvious the longer the couple have lived together. My married patients have often lived together for more than 50 years, and at this point I have sensed a "plasma" connecting them which, if broken by the death of one, often predicts the imminent death of the other.

Ronald and Judith had been married for 60 years. Ronald was an 86-year-old retired dentist, a veteran of World War Two and a cultured man with wide-ranging interests. Judith was 84 years old, a petite woman less than five feet tall and weighing only 90 lb. She had never worked professionally, but had donated her time and experience to many cultural and civic organizations. Ronald and Judith loved each other very much. On my first visit to them, I gave each of them a standard test for dementia, one part of which (designed to determine their facility with language) involves writing a simple sentence of their own choice. Each without the other's knowledge wrote "I love Judith" and "I love Ronald." The couple had had only one child but they had many grandchildren, whose pictures covered the walls of their center city apartment.

Both Ronald and Judith carried onerous chronic disease burdens, he with aortic stenosis, angina and gait dysfunction due to an old hip fracture, and she with polymyalgia rheumatica, emphysema, congestive heart failure, angina and a prior mitral valve replacement. Judith developed fever, anorexia and persistent weight loss (which she could ill afford). I asked her permission to admit her to hospital, but she refused, not wishing to leave her home or her husband. I obtained blood cultures and an echocardiogram in their home, and these suggested that endocarditis was the problem. I then started home infusion therapy of an antibiotic that could be delivered by Ronald just once per day, recognizing that it is just as important to protect the health of the caregiver as the health of the patient. Without the caregiver, the most carefully constructed plan of care will fall apart. In this instance, the preferable antibiotic would have been administered four times per day. "Second best" was a once-per-day drug, but this was much easier on Ronald. Judith initially responded to the drug, and her weight actually increased, although she never regained her original weight of 90 lb. Eventually she began a long, steady decline and died quietly at home, tended by the husband she loved so dearly. After her death, Ronald failed rapidly both physically and mentally, and died within ten months.

Margaret and Dorothy were spinster sisters who had lived together all their lives. Margaret was 92 and Dorothy was 90 years old. Both had hypertension and moderately severe dementia, but Margaret had emphysema whereas Dorothy had congestive heart failure and primary thrombocytosis. They lived alone in a Charles Adams-ish, antique-cluttered, dusty house dimly lit by a few incandescent bulbs. They had lived in that house together since they were little girls, and were now visited by their niece and nephew who did their shopping several times per week. The sisters were both frail, and vainly tried to remind each other to take their pills. When I visited them, one would say to the other "You're demented", and the other would respond with "No, you're demented!" They were adorable and touching in their tenderness and concern for each other. Dorothy died first, followed by Margaret within less than six months.

Giuseppe and Maria were an elderly Italian couple who had emigrated to the United States more than 60 years previously. They had never learned to speak English well, although Maria understood English. Giuseppe was 91 and Maria was 92 years old. They both had hypertension and hypothyroidism, but Giuseppe had had a recent stroke that had left him with aphasia and mild hemiparesis. They had one son with whom they were in daily phone contact, who visited them every weekend and who was always available when translation was absolutely necessary.

During the three years that I was their physician, I always saw them sitting in their living room, each in their own chair. Giuseppe was perennially skinny whereas Maria was quite ample. He was the more vocal of the two, but she always had the last word, often transmitted with a mere glance. Entering their home was a special treat. Their hospitality, warmth and genuine smiles of greeting were always the highlight of my day. Their devotion to each other was no less genuine. When Giuseppe died of a second stroke, Maria, although healthier than her husband, could not survive alone and died within three months of her husband's death, after a marriage of more than 70 years.

Unbroken Spirit

Many of my patients live under challenging conditions that often make me wonder how they survive, let alone thrive. But survive they do, and frequently with an unquenchable spirit that astonishes and elates me and reminds me daily why I so love what I do. Best of all, I am a part of their triumphs – sometimes an indispensable part, but always someone to whom they relate and with whom they share their feelings.

Edgar is a 75-year-old man who has severe congestive heart failure, hypertension, insulin-dependent diabetes mellitus and bilateral above-knee amputations. His wife, both of his parents and his only son have all died within the past three years. At my initial visit, Edgar had fluid in and around his lungs, and he also had fluid extending from his stumps to his chest wall. He was unable to wear his prostheses because they wouldn't fit over his waterlogged thighs. He slept on three pillows and was short of breath even at rest. His diabetes was poorly controlled and his salt intake was high.

I initiated treatment at home with large doses of diuretics, beta-blockers and ACE inhibitors, visited him three times per week and obtained frequent laboratory tests. I was also able to obtain electrocardiograms, chest X-rays and even echocardiograms in his home. When his shortness of breath did not resolve completely, I asked a hospital-based pulmonologist to remove fluid from around his lung. His shortness of breath then disappeared. I also instructed both Edgar and his sister-in-law (who bought his food) about dietary control of both diabetes and hypertension, by taking sample foods from his cupboards, refrigerator and freezer and going over their labeled carbohydrate and sodium contents, and explained to them how to stay within safe limits for both. After a few months of intensive home-based therapy for heart failure and diabetes control, Edgar was able to don his prostheses, and he now wears them all day. He goes up and down the stairs in his house and the stairs to the street. He goes to church every Sunday, goes out of the house regularly with friends, sleeps on one pillow, has installed manual controls in his car and is taking driving lessons at a local rehabilitation institute.

This story dramatically illustrates the value of evaluating and treating some patients at home. Most diagnostic tests are available at home. Clinical evaluation can be undertaken by frequent observation of a patient. If a patient doesn't have a caregiver, he or she must be sufficiently intelligent to know when to call for advice or assistance.

Sophie was a 95-year-old woman with hypertension, congestive heart failure, insulin-dependent diabetes mellitus and severe peripheral vascular disease. I had first met her four years previously, but within the following year she had lost both legs due to intractable pain. She was fitted with prostheses after each amputation, and bravely attended a rehabilitation institute for physical therapy to learn to walk. She was able to walk between bars with a physical therapist in attendance, but was unable to walk at home either independently or with assistance. Sophie became confined to either bed or a wheelchair. For transfers, personal cleanliness and meal preparation she was dependent on her daily home health aide and on her nephew, a Philadelphia policeman, who visited her three times per day, did her shopping and errands and apportioned her daily medications into a plastic pill sorter. Her hypertension was never adequately controlled, in part because she refused to take the diuretics that would rid her body of fluid, but only at the expense of keeping her soaked in urine for most of the day. She also stubbornly declined a catheter to keep her dry. As expected, she became progressively short of breath and eventually required three pillows to sleep comfortably. She died peacefully at home.

Sophie, despite her misfortunes, was always upbeat and a delight to talk to. She had many friends in her home on my frequent visits, and they were all invariably sunny and chatty. She would be taken from her home to attend church each Sunday by friends and church elders. Her god-daughter owned the most prominent funeral home in the area, and she often called me for an update on Sophie's condition. In short, Sophie was a vital and much loved member of her community, and her friends never let her forget that. She and I had a close relationship. She often asked me to call her because she "liked to hear my voice." When I told her that my chronic back problem was acting up, she would call me an "old man" and we would both laugh about it. Maybe Sophie was right! Perhaps I was in an "old man" frame of mind. Another of my nonagenarian patients once told me that 40 years previously he had decided that as long as he was able to stand, he would don his pants standing up – and he did! I often feel that these elderly people would not be prevented from enjoying life to the hilt by a stiff back and that, contrary to expectation, they have mentored me about how best to enjoy life.

Judy was a 62-year-old woman who had had two strokes due to hypertension, and lived in an upstairs bedroom where she was confined to either bed or a wheelchair. She had not been out of her bedroom in years. Her husband had died young, and she had raised six children alone while working as a cosmetologist. Two of her children were dead, another was in jail and two others had not communicated with her for years. Her last child, a daughter, was technically her caregiver and lived in her house, but in fact largely neglected her. On my visits, Judy's blood pressure might be either normal or astronomically high, depending on whether her daughter had picked up her medications from the pharmacy. I was able to solve at least that problem by switching her to a pharmacy that delivered her medications to her home. Meeting and talking to Judy would never have revealed her troubled and lonely life. She spent her days reading and listening to music. She never seemed to be bored and was certainly never boring. She was a fascinating conversationalist and was always upbeat and smiling. She died suddenly and alone. My entire office staff and I grieved for her, although I was the only one who had known her personally. Such was the force of Judy's personality.

Janet was a 74-year-old woman with aortic stenosis, rheumatoid arthritis, hypertension, diabetes mellitus, bilateral above-knee amputations, and a history of heart attack and left total hip replacement following a fall. She was of course bed-bound, but had an invariably sunny disposition. I remember her as if she were in front of me asking about my children and grandchildren by name, giving me small gifts for them and complimenting my wife for dressing me so nicely and taking good care of me. Janet's son called to tell me that she had died. I miss her still.

Louise was a 77-year-old woman with a long history of smoking and emphysema. I only knew her for two months, but she made an indelible impression on me. She was severely short of breath and needed to drink her nutrition because she didn't have the energy to chew. She was cared for by her husband of 56 years, a World War Two veteran who had participated in five European and African amphibious landings. The couple were very much in love. She did not have the breath to get out of bed, but he was always around her, talking to her and holding her. She was always perky and smiling. Louise and her husband told me how much they loved to dance together. My wife and I also enjoy dancing, and I talked with them about dancing even at my first visit.

When I first met Louise, it was apparent that she would die soon. Although it is rare for me to do so at the first visit, I introduced the subject of hospice care at that time. Both Louise and her husband needed no convincing, and immediately and gratefully seized upon the opportunity and asked me to make the appropriate arrangements. I did so, and visited Louise two more times before she died.

Marian, a 50-year-old woman, was my patient for six years. Over the years she became a friend to me, and much of my time with her was spent giving social advice and solace as well as hard medical advice. She had had polio as a child and had been wheelchair-bound for most of her life. She also had hypertension, a seizure disorder secondary to a stroke, and end-stage renal disease for which she had been on chronic hemodialysis since I first knew her. I met her when she lived in an apartment building run by the Department of Housing and Urban Development. The cinder block building was filthy, appearing from both without and within like a prison. I followed her to two more dwellings, the last of which was on the ground floor with a ramp leading to the front door for easy wheelchair access. About two years before she died, Marian fell from her wheelchair while transferring to her bed, suffered a severe fracture of her knee and underwent two arthroscopic surgeries and multiple courses of physical therapy sandwiched between her hemodialysis sessions. Through it all she maintained her equanimity, her control over her household and her watchfulness over her daughter and niece.

Marian confided in me about her 10-year-old daughter, who was bright and for whom she had tried unsuccessfully to get a scholarship to attend a private school in Philadelphia. Her niece, the daughter of her deceased sister, also lived with her. Marian had had a boyfriend for ten years who lived with her and took care of her basic needs when she was both well and ill. He looked after her daughter and niece when Marian was admitted to the hospital and when she went for dialysis. The two were close, and the daughter regarded him as her father, although he wasn't. About two years ago, the boyfriend took up with a younger woman who lived just a few doors down from Marian, and he moved out of her house. Marian was devastated by this betrayal, and for a month she was weepy and inconsolable. Gradually, she recovered from her loss and assumed a heightened self-respect. Although the boyfriend tried to resume his friendship with her, she refused to see him again or to allow him to come in her house or have any contact with her daughter or niece. To my surprise and delight, she told me how she had had an in-house date a few days earlier with the father-in-law of her home health aide. This man had been mugged and shot in the head several years previously but had made a good recovery with the exception of his speech, which was still indistinct but intelligible. Marian had sent her daughter and niece out to a neighbor's house during her date, explaining that "all girls needed privacy at such times." She said that she had had a "wonderful time" with him and that he was a "really nice man." The next day, he invited Marian and her daughter and niece to his family's Mother's Day outing, picked them up and brought them back. Once again she had a "wonderful time." I hadn't seen her so happy since I knew her, and was as pleased for her as if I had been a relative. During that relationship, Marian asked me to arrange a gynecological visit for her in preparation for sex with her new beau, and I was only too happy to do this.

Marian had a daily home health aide, and some of her needs were met by her daughter and niece. However, the majority of her daily needs were in the hands of her sister, whom Marian had invited to live with her and the girls free of charge in exchange for helping with the housekeeping. The sister indeed did this, but she was also a drug addict and frequently stole from Marian's slender supply of extra cash. As Marian's renal status deteriorated and the access sites for her dialysis shunts disappeared, she knew that she would soon have to make arrangements for the welfare of her daughter and her niece. She spoke to her father (her daughter's grandfather), who lived in Virginia, and he reassured her that he would take over the care of both girls should she die. I sent our social worker to her to give advice about writing a will to leave her meager estate to her daughter. Our social worker referred her to a lawyer, who accomplished this for a minimal fee. Within a few months, Marian had another seizure, aspirated and died in the hospital with pneumonia. Shortly after her death, her sister attempted to legally contest the will and seize her estate. Thanks to Marian's prudence and our social worker's watchfulness, she was unsuccessful. We still keep in contact with Marian's daughter and niece, and both are attending school and adjusting well to life with their grandfather in Virginia.

Unquenchable Responsibility to Family

Most of my medical training occurred in large city hospitals 35 to 40 years ago. At that time it was not uncommon to see elderly, infirm patients dropped off in an emergency room by family members without any history or background information. Often these family members would never return to see the patient, who would usually end their days in a nursing home. This practice was known among house officers as "dumping", and was universally regarded by us with loathing. As a young physician, it didn't occur to me that many of these families might have genuinely loved their elderly relatives. Unable to financially afford their care or to take on the responsibility of constantly staying with them when they needed to support their young children, they may have dropped them off at a city hospital knowing that they would at least be fed, clothed and housed.

When I became a consultant in gastroenterology in Tucson in 1970, patients were always referred to me by another physician. These patients and their families were closely knit, and the practice of "dumping" seemed to have disappeared. In retrospect, the major factor responsible for this was probably the enactment of Medicare and the rise of HMOs. These gave patients and their families the financial means to care for their loved ones without the shame or embarrassment of needing to accept charity. In addition, I found that certain ethnic groups were more culturally attuned to the care of their elderly. For example, Mexican-Americans rarely seemed to neglect their parents or indeed, relatives far more distant than parents. Asian-Americans also exhibited a fierce loyalty and obligation to the care of their elderly relatives. When I moved to Worcester, Norfolk and finally Philadelphia, I had the opportunity to observe how members of other ethnic groups care for their elderly, and I found that human attachments and commitments are the same across all races, ethnic groups and cultural backgrounds. I believe that people now know that elder care is a benefit for all citizens. They do not need to beg or grovel for humane treatment.

Having said that, there are exceptionally memorable instances of exceptional care for family members that I would like to cite because they are illustrative of extraordinary sacrifices that often go unnoticed.

Robert is a 52-year-old man with the unenviable chronic disease burden of hypertension, insulin-dependent diabetes mellitus with peripheral neuropathy, chronic bilateral lower extremity cellulitis and symptomatic prostatic enlargement. Two years ago, he sustained a large myocardial infarction with resultant severe congestive heart failure. He has been virtually immobile due to a combination of heart failure (shortness of breath) and chronic venous disease with skin breakdown. Robert never married. However, his younger brother (who is married with children and holds a full-time job) visits him daily, before going to work in the morning and on the way back from work at night. He shops for Robert, prepares his food, places his many medicines in a pill sorter, cleans the house, does the laundry and performs errands. He also arranges for food stamps and help from other social service agencies for his brother.

I started diuretics and other medications for congestive heart failure, initiated insulin therapy and procured a diabetes education nurse to teach Robert and his brother about insulin injections, blood sugar measurements and how to shop for and prepare a diabetic and low-salt diet. I also obtained a wound care nurse, started chronic antibiotic therapy for Robert's cellulitis, and started medication to relieve his urinary bladder outlet obstruction. Within six weeks, his blood sugars were under excellent control, he was able to climb a flight of stairs in his house without stopping to rest, the open sores on his legs had healed and he was urinating normally. However, none of this would have been possible without the devotion, cooperation and sacrifice of his brother. I have told Robert's brother many times that he is saintly, a comment that he shrugs off as unnecessary praise.

Betty is an 80-year-old woman who gave birth to a son out of wedlock at the age of 17 years. This child was born with cerebral palsy and is unable to speak, although he understands simple directions. He has considerable muscle spasticity and spends his life either sitting or lying on a bed or sitting on a commode. In addition to his birth defect, he also has hypertension, non-insulin-dependent diabetes and chronic ulcerative colitis. Betty subsequently married and had several other children, all of whom are now grown. Her children and grandchildren are all loyal to her and adore her. As matriarch of the family, she holds Sunday dinners at her home which are always well attended and which she prepares herself.

However, Betty lives alone with her now 63-year-old son and takes care of him by herself (although she has offers of help from her granddaughters). She sleeps in the same room with him, prepares his meals, does his laundry, gives him his medicines and provides him with all the support that such a chronically disadvantaged person requires, although she herself has hypertension and coronary artery disease. Betty has done an extraordinary job of taking meticulous care of her son while successfully raising the rest of her family.

Len and Pam, aged 80 and 78 years, respectively, had been married for almost 60 years. They were both moderately demented, but in addition Len had chronic lung disease and congestive heart failure while Pam had hypertension, atrial fibrillation and non-insulin-dependent diabetes mellitus. They lived in a second-floor bedroom of a house that was actually owned and maintained by their son, an only child. The couple had poor mobility, so their son hired attendants to prepare their food and sit with them in shifts, feed them and take care of their bodily needs. The son worked in construction, traveled to New York City every night during the week to work, rode back on the train each morning to Philadelphia, slept briefly and then visited his parents and, if necessary, would take them to a consultant, emergency room or X-ray facility. If either of his parents needed hospitalization, he found time to visit them daily and to thoroughly question any specialist on the case. He also managed to take care of his wife, who has rheumatoid arthritis.

Throughout the two years that I knew and cared for Len and Pam, I repeatedly presented to their son the advantages and benefits of placing his parents in a nursing home, a recommendation that I rarely make and never make lightly. He understood the relief of stress in his life that a nursing home placement would bring, but refused to consider it. Len died first, during a hospitalization for septic arthritis. Pam, barely able to comprehend that her husband had passed away, died a few months later at her son's home under hospice care. Her son called me several days later to thank me for all the support that I had given him. In truth, my contribution to the support of his parents seemed minuscule compared with his monumental effort.

Occasionally, I have seen devoted care delivered for long periods by a person completely unrelated to the patient. My most memorable example of this occurred as the result of a deathbed promise.

Ellen was an 81-year-old woman with a history of progressive and severe dementia for at least five years. Her only child, a 50-year-old man, had been her caregiver but had died three years previously. However, before he died, his girlfriend had promised him that she would take care of his mom when he was unable to do so – *and she did!* She lived with the bed-bound, totally immobile and uncommunicative Ellen for three years, fed, bathed and changed her, shifted her position in bed several times per day to prevent bed sores, and rarely left the house until Ellen died.

Lisa is a 75-year-old woman who is a bed-bound invalid. The cause of her condition is obscure. She had been evaluated repeatedly for eight years before I took on her care for vague and debilitating abdominal pains. When she had been ambulatory, she had had all the appropriate tests and procedures to uncover the reason for her complaints, but none had ever been found. When I became her physician, she was confined to an upstairs bedroom and was totally dependent on care, including feeding. However, she was able to speak and answer questions intelligently, although her conversational ability was limited. In addition, she had insulin-dependent diabetes mellitus, hypertension and hypothyroidism, all of which were well controlled.

Lisa had been married for more than 50 years to Don, her childhood sweetheart. The couple had been unable to have children, but they adopted fraternal twins (a boy and girl, now 39 years old) who visited them frequently. Don was 80 years old but appeared no older than 65. He was a physically powerful man with an equally powerful and ebullient personality. However, when tending to his wife, he was the essence of tenderness, speaking to her softly and handling her efficiently but delicately. Don was Lisa's sole caregiver. They had a home health aide and visiting nurse furnished by PCA, but Don was jealous of his prerogatives and allowed the aide only minimal household duties, while he handled the majority of chores pertaining to his wife.

I loved visiting Lisa and Don, and especially talking to Don. He was a veteran of World War Two and had served in the famed

82nd Airborne Division at the Battle of the Bulge. He would recall to me the ferocity of that fight and his buddies who had died there. After the war, he became a bus driver for the city of Philadelphia, retiring on social security and a small pension. Don always dominated any conversation. Proud of his physique and his physical abilities, he would playfully challenge and box with me. However, even when talking with me, he might remember something he had forgotten to do for his wife, and would rush off to attend to it and be with her.

Don was a healthy man with the exception of a long history of depression and slash marks on his wrists to prove it. He was under the long-term care of a psychiatrist at the Veterans' Administration Hospital. Whenever I asked him how he felt, his answer would be "Great!" However, he had recently begun to tell me that he was feeling "weary and exhausted." But no matter how tired he felt, it was clear that he would never consider a nursing home placement for his wife.

I didn't expect the call I received one morning from his daughter telling me that she had found her father dead in bed. My first thought was that he had committed suicide. The medical examiner ordered a post-mortem examination but found that, although he had no history of cardiac disease, Don had died of a heart attack. No evidence of medication- or toxin-induced death was discovered. The couple's children were in a quandary. Although it was clear that Lisa would now require a nursing home placement and that they would need to watch their mother 24/7 until that was obtained, they had no idea how to carry out the duties that Don had performed with such apparent efficiency and ease.

At once I called PCA and explained the situation. With their characteristic empathy and efficiency they arrived on the scene within an hour, patiently explained to the anxious children what they would need to do for the next few days, and then arranged for Lisa's admission to a nursing home within 48 hours. (In the interim, I also called Don's psychiatrist at the VA Hospital to tell him that Don's death had not been due to suicide.)

Although I have seen many examples of close family bonding and exemplary care given to elderly patients, I also want to describe a patient who was treated with total contempt by her family. Carol was a 66-year-old woman with hypertension,

insulin-dependent diabetes mellitus, rheumatoid arthritis, hypothyroidism and severe gastroesophageal disease. She was able to
stand with difficulty, and could walk with the aid of a platform
walker which I had procured for her. I was able to control her
hypertension, blood sugars, thyroid function and heartburn, but
was unable to stimulate any sense of responsibility among her
family for her care. Reproduced below is the last letter of consultation that I wrote for Carol to her primary physician.

Dear Dr. ...,
I saw Carol again on December 16, 2002. She is profoundly
depressed and for good reason. About 4–5 months ago, her
daughter who lives with her suggested that she should ''go into
a home.'' Since then this daughter has mentioned it with
increasing frequency, and Carol's sister and her other daughter
who lives in Florida have given her similar advice. Carol,
weeping, said that she had always worked hard and that she
would never go into a home. She also said that she would never
have placed her own mother in a home. Carol gets no help for
any of her basic needs, although her house is literally overrun
with teenage grandchildren. She has no privacy because her bed
(out of which she can barely move) lies just inside the front door.
Even when she uses the commode, she is in full view of everyone.
Her husband has severe emphysema and never ventures out of a
small alcove on the first floor. The daughter who lives with her
was taken to the hospital two days ago with uncontrolled
diabetes and was immediately transferred to the ICU with
pulmonary edema (and a possible heart attack). Carol was
just released from ... Hospital for evaluation of the neck pain to
which I alluded in my last letter to you. No cause of that pain
was found, but the severity was considerably relieved. Since
discharge, she had not adhered to a diabetic/low-salt diet and
had not recently taken her blood sugars. I cannot vouch that she
has taken her medications regularly. Incidentally, I asked her
whether she had considered suicide, and her answer was ''yes.''
However, she does not have a plan for suicide, nor has she ever
made an attempt.

PE: Patient is depressed and crying. Lies flat comfortably. She
can rise to a sitting position only with great effort and dis-
comfort, and is unable to stand. Vermin share her bed with her.

BP – 165/105 (LA, sit) AR – 84, reg
Lungs, Heart – no change from my last letter.
Ext – bilateral 2–3 + pedal/pretibial edema.

Impression – Dr. ..., Carol requires an acute intervention involving help for her creature comfort needs, psychiatric and/ or medicinal help for depression, and motivation to continue her diabetic and anti-hypertensive treatments. Paula [her case manager] and I have already discussed the options, and none of them sounds optimal. I started her on sertraline [an anti-depressant] 50 mg qd, but Carol probably doesn't have the money to purchase it long term. She should really be extracted from that hellish environment, but this sounds like ''the home'' to which she said she'd never move. I have sent a social worker to see Carol who is working with PCA to either get her substantive help or place her in a facility where she will get the help that she so desperately needs. With your permission, I would like to sign any necessary papers to assure expedited removal from her environment.

Sincerely,
Alfred E. Stillman, MD, MACP

Shortly after this letter was written, Carol was hospitalized emergently with dyspnea and died in hospital.

"But She Has Such a Pretty Face"

How often have we heard that terse back-handed compliment glibly applied to a more detailed but unflattering description of a fat person? The patients of whom I speak and for whose general health I am responsible are not plump or portly – they are fat, and morbidly so. They are usually middle-aged women whose weight ranges from 350 to 600 lb, and their obesity not only limits their mobility but also imposes a long list of chronic medical complications on their already difficult lives. These people commonly have a strong family history of obesity and were frequently "the largest kid in the class", even in elementary school. As they became more obese, especially in their teen and young adult years, they may have become socially isolated due to a combination of their decreased ability to play sports or even ambulate, their rejection by schoolmates who were societally obsessed with being thin, and their increasingly poor self-image. Moreover, if in order to leave their home to visit a physician they require a special stretcher manned by two full teams of emergency medical technicians, even simple medical problems may pose a life-threatening dilemma unless a doctor visits them in their home. By the time these patients have been referred to us (usually by visiting nurses), they are likely to have unsuccessfully rotated through multiple diets and entrepreneurial weight loss schemes, and may not have seen a physician in years.

As we know, morbidly obese patients often have medical conditions incited and fueled by their habitus. The more common of these are listed below.

- Hypertension – already a serious risk for cardiovascular, cerebrovascular and renal disease in the person of normal body habitus, but morbid obesity magnifies these risks by rendering blood pressure more difficult to measure reliably and by adding to the workload on the heart. Hypertension in the morbidly obese person must be treated particularly aggressively.
- Glucose intolerance – the tissues of the morbidly obese person are relatively resistant to the effect of insulin. Therefore, in these individuals, in order to maintain a normal blood glucose, the pancreas must continually produce a larger amount of insulin than the pancreas of a thin person. Obese people can

maintain a normal blood glucose, but only at the risk of eventually exhausting their pancreas. Should this occur, the patient will develop frank diabetes mellitus. To delay this event, we need to give the patient medication to increase the peripheral sensitivity of their tissues to insulin and/or to supply extra insulin by injection, and to educate them with regard to the value of a diabetic-type diet. Vigorous exercise, a modality commonly used to help control blood sugars in mobile individuals, is not applicable to morbidly obese patients.

- Obstructive sleep apnea – this condition is characterized by inappropriate daytime sleepiness and prominent nocturnal snoring. Although often associated with morbid obesity, it can also occur in individuals of normal habitus. It is caused by transient airway collapse that results in multiple episodes of interrupted sleep of which the patient is unaware. It can cause low blood oxygen levels during sleep and hypertension in blood vessels of the lung and periphery, leading to congestive heart failure. Obstructive sleep apnea can be confirmed by physiologically monitoring the patient during a nocturnal sleep study. Treatment is usually administered by having the patient sleep while wearing a device that prevents the airways from collapsing during sleep. Getting the morbidly obese patient to a sleep center can be both physically and administratively demanding.

- Degenerative joint disease – this medical condition is often familiarly referred to when communicating with lay persons as "wear and tear arthritis." It commonly, although not exclusively, affects the body's weight-bearing joints (hips, knees, ankles and vertebrae), and is understandably more severe in individuals who are extremely overweight. Arthritic pain is usually treated with medications to relieve pain or inflammation. Joint replacement surgery is generally not an option for morbidly obese patients unless they can first lose a significant amount of weight, which is too difficult a goal for most of these patients to achieve.

- Deconditioning – this medical term refers to muscle weakness secondary to prolonged disuse. Immobility produced by a combination of morbid obesity and deconditioning fosters spiraling loss of muscle function. Morbidly obese patients lose mobility because their muscles are too weak to support their weight, or their heart or lungs cannot send sufficient blood or oxygen to their muscles to allow this exertion, or because they are afraid of falling. Restoring their muscular tone requires a large reduction in weight, prolonged physical therapy and, frequently, psychological support to bolster their confidence.

- Functional incontinence – this occurs when, despite normal function of the patient's bladder or rectum, they cannot reach the toilet sufficiently quickly to avoid wetting or soiling themselves. Fear of becoming a public spectacle often keeps them from socializing or even venturing out of their home or apartment. This type of incontinence can usually be helped by frequent toileting or by using a bedside or conveniently placed commode. However, these solutions often continue to chain the patient to their home.
- Depression – this is an understandable and frequent consequence for patients who have often done their best to reduce weight without noticeable effect, have limited contact with other people and have a poor self-image. Their lives are often spent in bed or alternating between bed and a large chair in which they may sit for the majority of the day without moving. They are frequently totally dependent on caregivers. Although they can feed themselves independently, they require help to dress or bathe, to empty their commode or get to a bathroom, and to walk or transfer from one location to another (these five activities are collectively referred to as *activities of daily living*, and are the most basic functional requirements for living). Moreover, they are often unable to perform the small tasks that being part of a household community involves (e.g. shopping, cooking, cleaning the house, doing laundry, etc.), which further demeans them. It is no small wonder that many of these patients are depressed and may require long-term medication for relief.

Finally, morbid obesity places patients at high risk for emergency and even elective surgical procedures. Standard hospital beds, stretchers, X-ray tables and CT/MRI scanners are often inadequate to safely and comfortably support or house their bulk. The risk of complications (e.g. ICU admission, post-operative ventilation, venous clots and pulmonary embolization, pneumonia, etc.) during the post-operative period for any procedure that requires general anesthesia and bed rest is considerable, and often necessitates special screening tests to ensure that these patients can safely undergo the ordeal. Bariatric surgery, often the last hope for reducing the morbidly obese to a safer body mass, will not be performed unless the surgeon is assured that his patient has been approved for surgery by psychiatric, metabolic, cardiopulmonary and dietary consultants, and that the risk of operation is less than that of not operating.

Three case histories of morbidly obese patients follow. Each of these patients has had their own serious habitus-related complications, but their courses have taken very different turns.

Steve is a 53-year-old man whose downward medical spiral began in 1991. Until then, with the exception of inadequately treated hypertension, he had been a healthy, fit and powerful person. He had attended college in North Carolina, where he had been a member of his college fencing (saber) team and had majored in law enforcement and criminology. After graduation, he worked on the administrative staff of a local Philadelphia prison. He married a schoolteacher and had three sons, all of whom were college graduates. He adored his grandchildren and always bragged about them.

However, between 1991 and 1997 Steve suffered three strokes, the last of which was the most severe. Indeed, he had made significant recoveries after the initial two strokes and had continued to work. After the last stroke he never worked or walked again, and he became bed-bound, although he retained all of his considerable cognitive abilities and hand function, and he remained continent. During his last stroke-related hospital and rehab unit stay, despite anticoagulant therapy, he developed blood clots in both legs and pulmonary emboli. A filter was placed in the main vein of his body to prevent recurrence. This maneuver was successful in protecting his lungs, but resulted in further massive clot formation in both legs up to the level of the filter. Steve's continued inactivity and bed rest combined with a huge appetite as a consequence of boredom resulted in his gaining weight. (When a homebound and bed-bound patient develops morbid obesity, it is difficult to obtain a reliable weight or keep track of it on a frequent basis. Only bariatric units in hospitals have sufficiently accurate scales to do the job. Otherwise these people, even in a hospital, are often weighed on commercial cargo scales in a kitchen used to weigh sides of beef.)

When I took over Steve's care in 2000, I met a hugely obese man with grotesquely swollen legs who appeared to ooze over the bed like an ameba, but who was articulate and upbeat. His wife worked six days per week, and began her daily duties taking care of him in the late afternoon as soon as she returned from her job. The couple's sons tried to look in on him when their mother was working. Steve always set long-term goals and dates for himself, which he shared with his family and me, by which times he promised that he would be able to walk. He told me that his son was getting married in one year and that he expected to take him down the aisle on his feet. On another occasion, he looked forward to the birth of a grandchild in six months' time and expected to coo over the baby's crib on his own feet standing to his full height. Neither of these expectations (or several other similar ones) was ever realized, but certainly not due to lack of effort on Steve's part. Despite my better judgment about his negligible ambulatory potential, Steve so inspired me to help him realize his dreams that I obtained physical therapists for him at home and, after much hard negotiation with his HMO, admitted him for three weeks to a rehab unit. He worked bravely and hard but was unable to stand up. In fact, he was unable to sit up without assistance or even to turn from side to side in bed independently (the most basic mobility skill).

During my five years as Steve's physician, he developed virtually every serious complication of morbid obesity. After his wife told me of his loud snoring, I arranged evaluation for obstructive sleep apnea, which of course he had. He had also developed pulmonary (in addition to his prior systemic) hypertension punctuated by periodic episodes of congestive heart failure. His blood sugars also rose, requiring treatment with medication and dietary education. Although Steve had always been meticulous about his appearance and cleanliness, even when bed bound, prolonged immobility and the absence during much of the day of anyone to take care of his bodily needs eventually resulted in his complete incontinence. This in turn was followed by multiple festering, painful pressure ulcers which were most difficult to visualize and dress because they lay on the undersurface of a man weighing at least 500 lb. Two bariatric surgeons refused to operate on him because of his chronic disease load.

Steve continued to take an anticoagulant (warfarin) to limit further clot proliferation. After he had been taking warfarin for several years, he developed massive rectal bleeding for which he was rushed to the hospital with his usual complement of two full teams of emergency medical technicians. Efforts to uncover the source of this life-threatening bleed (e.g. upper and lower gastrointestinal endoscopy, nuclear medicine study, X-rays of abdominal vessels) were unsuccessful largely due to his bulk. Needless to say, no surgeon wanted to operate on him. His hemorrhage eventually required 12 units of blood transfusion over two days, at the end of which the bleeding mercifully stopped spontaneously. Steve never again had warfarin and never again bled from his gastrointestinal tract.

As the years passed, Steve realized that he would never walk again. His bubbly personality turned to depression. After months of antidepressant medication and visits by psychiatric nurses and social workers, he told me that he would like to undergo amputation of both his legs, thereby removing the most ponderous part of his body and allowing him to take advantage of his upper body strength so that he might sit in a wheelchair and move around his house, visit his family and be less of a burden to his wife. He and I realized that this was a major psychological change from hopeful fantasy to a realistic assessment of goals and how to achieve them. Once again I negotiated with Steve's HMO to allow psychiatric, surgical and physiatric (rehabilitation medicine) consultations to be performed in a single day with the aim of performing bilateral leg amputations to increase his mobility and decrease his dependency. As a preliminary step, I asked the HMO to allow a CT scan to determine the extent of clot in his legs, and they agreed to this. When I was finally able to locate a CT scanner large enough to accommodate Steve, and to transport him there, the radiologist reported that clot was present throughout his venous system up to the filter that had been placed so many years before. Although this might have meant amputation at the level of the hips, Steve agreed and looked forward to semi-independence.

At this point, his wife was hospitalized with a heart attack and Steve developed depression to the point of considering suicide. With his wife sick and no longer able to give him the attention he required, and with his recent and rapid affective transitions from unrealistic, blissful hopefulness through grimly coming to terms with reality and finally contemplating suicide, Steve and his wife reluctantly agreed to his placement in a nursing home. The family had been forced into making this decision by Steve's multiple illnesses, primary among them morbid obesity, his wife's recent cardiac incapacitation, and their HMO, which had reached the limit of any further expenditures that they would make on Steve's behalf at home.

Marilyn is a 68-year-old woman with a lifelong history of obesity. As she explained it to me seven years ago, her birth weight was 15 lb. She was always the largest girl in her class, and by the age of 13 years she weighed 200 lb. Her mother, daughter and granddaughter are all obese, although not to the same degree as Marilyn. Two of her younger obese sisters have died during the seven years during which I have been her physician. Marilyn's daughter and granddaughter live with her, and they and a home health aide provided by her Medicaid HMO handle her basic physical needs. She eats independently and is functionally incontinent. She relies on her aide to bathe her and change her nightgown. However, she makes and receives telephone calls, takes her own medications and pays her own bills.

Marilyn had been diagnosed with obstructive sleep apnea two years before I became her physician. She was treated with the appropriate equipment, but was unable to tolerate the discomfort associated with its use (a not uncommon finding in these patients). She had also been diagnosed with moderately severe asthma, and was taking many medications for relief of wheezing, including atomized steroids and bronchodilators, into her airways. However, review of her history also revealed that she had symptomatic gastroesophageal reflux (which may frequently provoke reflex bronchoconstriction). Trial initiation of a powerful inhibitor of gastric acid production combined with elimination of asthma medications (including theophylline, which weakens the gastroesophageal barrier and promotes reflux) resulted in complete relief of wheezing. Marilyn has not needed asthmatic medications for three years.

My estimate of Marilyn's weight is close to 600 lb. Although she had been able to ambulate gingerly with the help of a rolling walker and under constant surveillance, she took to her bed permanently two years before I first met her, due to a combination of morbid obesity, muscular weakness and pulmonary difficulties. When I first visited her, as with so many similar patients, she insisted that she would walk again. I obtained physical therapists for her, and she was able to sit up independently but was never capable of moving off her bed safely. A few years ago, after continued bed confinement and intermittent home physical therapy for five years, Marilyn became depressed and needed medication for rescue. She is insured by a Medicaid HMO, and it is extremely unlikely that she will be afforded the chance to have bariatric surgery and all the pre- and post-operative evaluations that that would entail. Now resigned to spending the rest of her life in bed, she is emotionally stable and takes an active role in guiding and mentoring her granddaughter. She is the matriarch of her family, but would certainly prefer less reverence and more mobility.

Shelly is a 47-year-old woman with morbid obesity, obstructive sleep apnea and hypertension. In addition, she has chronic bronchitis secondary to long-term tobacco abuse. Her parents are deceased. She never married, but has a 26-year-old son whom she sees three times per week. She lives with her two sisters (aged 45 and 50 years) who are her primary caregivers. She had last worked as a school aide 14 years before I first saw her.

I first met Shelly two years ago, in winter. Her home was freezing, dark and filthy. Shelly was filthy as well. Her home had space heaters but these were either not turned on or not working. She was lying on her bed just inside the front entrance of her home. The only light in the large room was obtained when a sister stood on a rickety chair and screwed in a low-wattage incandescent bulb. At that first visit, Shelly had not walked for two years and was unable to transfer, even with assistance, to a commode. Consequently, all her activities of daily living (eating, bathing, changing clothes, defecation and urination) were conducted within the narrow confines of her bed.

When I initially examined Shelly, her blood pressure was 175/110 and she was devouring a large bag of salty potato chips. She had a cavernous wound in her left upper thigh that was draining blood and pus. I immediately arranged for hospitalization, fearing that she had either a huge pressure ulcer or a fistula. A brief hospital stay revealed the wound to be a pressure ulcer. I had felt that Shelly would do best in a convalescent center where she would be certain to receive her medications, appropriate wound care and dietary instruction to at least initiate weight reduction. However, Shelly was found to be fully capable of making her own decisions, including those regarding her health, and she insisted on going home. The hospital and staff were legally and ethically bound to honor her wishes, so Shelly was returned to her home and sisters. I continued to visit her at home, and after prolonged antibiotic therapy and frequent visits by wound care nurses, the wound completely closed. Meanwhile, I normalized Shelly's blood pressure and, although she was not frankly diabetic, began medication to improve her sensitivity to insulin and relieve metabolic stress on her pancreas.

Six months later, Shelly contracted pneumonia and I sent her to the hospital. This was uneventfully cured but, instead of another discharge back home, I managed to have her admitted to a newly opened bariatric unit at a rehabilitation hospital in Philadelphia. She stayed there for six weeks and lost 47 lb on an 1800-calorie, low-sodium diet. She also had daily physical therapy, and at discharge was able to stand and ambulate for short distances with a rolling walker. Her blood pressure on discharge was 125/80.

When I now visit Shelly at home, I find her eating lunch consisting of a salad and fresh fruit. She has not reverted to her previous dietary habits or cigarettes and, with continued physical therapy at home, continues to make progress with her mobility. She also maintains regular contact with her bariatrician, and is being considered for bariatric surgery. Shelly has shown that she has the will and the perseverance to work towards a difficult goal. Ultimately, the investment in this patient, should she undergo successful surgery, will be amply repaid by restoring her sense of personal worth and her independent position in her family and society, reinvigorating her physicians and therapists to extend their efforts to other morbidly obese patients, and saving society many thousands of dollars that would otherwise have been spent on Shelly's future care.

Neuromuscular Disease

Imagine a person – young, fully active and filled with antici-
pation of future parties, romances, friends to meet, schools
to attend, careers to begin, babies to hold, wives, husbands or
significant others to kiss, dreams to realize – whose life is changed
by diving head first into shallow water or some similar sudden
unexpected trauma. Or imagine another person, slightly older than
the first, who has already settled into a comfortable lifestyle but
who notices the gradual onset of strange bodily sensations or
clumsiness, frightening him into a physician's office where, after
tests and consultations, he is given bad news. Or imagine a young
woman, married and working, who gives birth to a child with
cerebral palsy, mental retardation or genetic disease that results
not only in the dedication of her entire future to the child's care,
but also to the destruction of her family and support systems and
her isolation from normal social activity.

Young or middle-aged people with severe neuromuscular
disease are largely immobile and consequently share several
problems with the morbidly obese (e.g. depression, incontinence, deconditioning), but the more profound immobility affecting the former often leads to a more progressive and
relentless course. Moreover, each of the different types of neuromuscular disease has its own side-effects depending on the part
of the nervous system that is affected.

The brain controls bodily functions by either manufacturing
hormones that affect distant parts of the body (or other areas of
the brain itself) or by passing electrical impulses into the spinal
cord (the extension of the brain protected by the spine or
vertebral column). Peripheral nerves emanate from the spinal
cord throughout its length and ramify over the entire body,
conducting the brain's messages to distant sites.

Quadriplegia occurs if the spinal cord is traumatized or severed
in the neck. The peripheral nerves that govern movement of the
legs leave the cord in the low back, while those that dictate arm
and hand movement leave the cord between the fifth cervical
(neck) and the first thoracic (chest) vertebrae. Any severe damage to the spinal cord at this level will produce leg paralysis, while
the degree of upper extremity paralysis will depend on how
many of the cervical nerves still maintain their connection with
the brain. In addition, peripheral nerves not only conduct impulses for movement from the brain to muscles, but also conduct

sensory impulses in the opposite direction, warning the brain of unpleasant or dangerous sensations (e.g. heat, sharp objects or an incipient fall). For example, a spinal fracture at the fourth cervical vertebra would produce total paralysis of and absent sensation in the arms and hands, while a fracture at the eighth cervical vertebra would still allow significant motion and sensation in those organs. Because of their inability to perceive noxious sensations below the level of cord injury, such patients are at high risk of and may be unable to avoid serious injuries.

In addition to impaired extremity motion and sensation, cord injury at any level also profoundly affects bladder and bowel function and sexual satisfaction and performance.

- The urinary bladder distends with huge volumes of urine which the patient cannot completely empty under voluntary control, and which serve as a breeding ground for urinary tract infection. Control of continence and potential urinary sepsis necessitates bladder catheterization, which itself carries a risk of urinary tract infection. If the patient has the use of his hands, intermittent self-catheterization should be optimally performed three to four times per day. If the patient is quadriplegic and cannot use his hands, an indwelling bladder catheter draining into a plastic bag will be needed. Catheterized patients should have yearly imaging of their urinary tract to monitor possible development of stones or cancer (to which prolonged bladder catheterization predisposes).
- Cord injury at any level will also cause lower bowel and rectal distension, requiring lifelong dependence on stool softeners, suppositories, enemas or digital fecal disimpaction.
- An important set of nerves (the sympathetic nervous system) flows down the cord from the brain and exits the cord at all 12 thoracic vertebrae and the first several lumbar (low back) vertebrae. If cord interruption occurs above the first thoracic vertebra, the sympathetic nervous system will not be able to reach crucial organs such as the heart, blood vessels, lungs, intestine, kidneys, urinary bladder and many intra-abdominal glands. Decreased sympathetic innervation may cause blood pressure instability and autonomic dysreflexia manifested as extreme hypertension and other symptoms in response to

noxious stimuli (usually excessive bladder or bowel distension). Moreover, the sympathetic nervous system also me-
diates sweating. On a hot day, the normal person eliminates
excess body heat by sweating, but the quadriplegic, who is
unable to perspire, will require fans, air conditioners and fluid
replacement.

- Penile erection occurs via cerebral (visual, remembered or
imagined) or tactile stimulation. The former stimuli are the
more effective methods, but these are compromised when the
connection between brain and spinal cord is severed. However, tactile stimulation of the penis can still achieve erection,
and addition of oral medications such as sildenafil, injection of
certain amines into the base of the penis and insertion of
penile tumescent pumps can allow erection and intercourse.
Cord-injured women may experience decreased vaginal secretions and difficult (although not painful) intercourse, but
this can be relieved with the application of vaginal lubricants.

The diaphragm – the main muscle of respiration, which separates
the chest from the abdomen – is innervated by the third, fourth
and fifth cervical nerves. The effect of a high cord injury on a
patient's ability to breathe will depend on how many of these
three peripheral nerves maintain their connection to the brain. A
patient with a cord injury at C3 or higher will need a respirator in
order to survive.

The immobilized patient, whether their immobility is due to
spinal cord injury, multiple sclerosis or severe Parkinson's disease, is at risk for multiple pressure ulcers. Such ulcers may
become quite deep, penetrating even to underlying bone, or may
become infected, acting as a source of sepsis. Pressure ulcers will
occur unless the patient's body position is rotated every few
hours to prevent prolonged contact with the surface on which
they are lying leading to decreased skin blood flow and injury. If
their skin integrity is jeopardized by dragging them across the
sheets or other surfaces, producing skin tears, these minor
breaches may become major entry points for bacteria into the
interior of the body. The skin of these patients must be routinely
and meticulously examined for the earliest signs of injury. They
should also lie on special mattresses designed to decrease the
pressure on their skin, and their nutrition must be bolstered so

that they will have the protein reserves necessary to repair a wound should one occur. Because sensation may be impaired (at least in individuals with cord injury or multiple sclerosis), the patient will be unable to assist in pressure ulcer detection or tell us whether they are experiencing discomfort. Therefore it is the caregivers' responsibility to prevent pressure ulcers in these patients.

Patients who spend all of their time in bed and indoors can also expect dissolution of bone when, due to lack of weight bearing, their bones "forget their purpose." Lack of exposure to sunlight reduces vitamin D production (the activated form of vitamin D is manufactured in the skin and is mediated by ultraviolet rays, but window glass filters out these rays). This predisposes such patients to fractures following even minor trauma, and to kidney stones as the calcium from their bones is lost in their urine or may precipitate in their urinary tract. Indeed, 30% of a patient's bone loss occurs in the first six months following paralysis. These bony metabolic problems can often be delayed or mollified by administration of vitamin D and other medications (e.g. bisphosphonates) to prevent the body's natural process of bone destruction.

Although cord-severed patients cannot feel externally delivered sensation below the level of injury, they may experience neuropathic pain which the injured nerves themselves generate. This pain always occurs below the level of injury, most commonly in the hands or feet, and is described by the patient as "burning." The immobile limbs are also subject to spasms and, due to increased muscle tone, to contractures. Contraction of a leg at the knee, if uncorrected, might prevent the patient from sitting on a chair. The same process at the ankle would prevent the patient from wearing a shoe. Fortunately, both neuropathic pain and spasms can be treated with medication. Contractures must be prevented by stretching the affected limbs daily to their full range of motion. Once an established contracture has occurred, only orthopedic procedures (e.g. surgery or progressive casting) will suffice to restore the limb to a functional position.

In patients with multiple sclerosis there is random destruction of neural protective sheaths (myelin) throughout the nervous system. They too are at risk of falling due to muscular weakness and clumsiness as well as an impaired sense of balance and vision. In individuals with Parkinson's disease there is damage to particular brain sites that are important for maintaining muscular flexibility and tone. Because of their muscular rigidity and dysfunction and a special propensity to develop dementia, they are at high risk for falls and aspiration pneumonia. Falls, particularly in thin individuals, are especially liable to result in hip, wrist, vertebral and other fractures, while aspiration of stomach food contents and acid produces infectious and chemical damage to the lungs.

Joseph is a 68-year-old man who suddenly became paraplegic about six years ago due to an unsuspected spinal infection. He underwent emergency lumbar spine surgery without neurological improvement. Prior to surgery, Joseph had been able to walk and work, but since surgery he has not walked again and has been bed-bound. Between six and nine months following surgery, he developed progressive weakness and eventual paralysis of his right arm, the cause of which was never discovered. He also has a formidable chronic disease load, including hypertension, insulin-dependent diabetes mellitus, arteriosclerotic heart disease (with prior heart attack), peripheral arterial disease (for which he had undergone an arterial bypass to divert blood to his legs), psoriasis, and a history of venous clots and pulmonary emboli (sustained following spinal surgery, and for which he had placement of a venous filter).

Joseph has been married to his present wife for the past 27 years. She is his sole and devoted caregiver, and has had no assistance from home health aides. The couple live with a 24-year-old daughter and a baby granddaughter, on whom Joseph dotes. Joseph eats independently but is dependent for all other activities of daily living, and wears a bladder catheter. He has a prickly, pugnacious personality and unleashes it on anyone in the vicinity, including his wife and myself (but never his granddaughter). His visiting nurse, his wife and I have always thought that he was capable of transferring with assistance to a wheelchair, but he has always vociferously turned down this suggestion.

I have been Joseph's physician for the past three and a half years. He belongs to an HMO and has a physician who has been assigned to him but whom, as so often happens with bed-bound patients, he has not seen in years. The HMO designates me as a home-visit consultant, and the HMO physician of record is only too happy to allow me to order medications and routine tests. For my part, I send the HMO doctor a descriptive letter every time I see "his" patient, outlining the patient's status and my reasons for altering therapies. Should I need to hospitalize the patient or order an unusual test (some HMOs regard a simple chest X-ray as "unusual"), I must first obtain the permission of the physician of record. During my relationship with Joseph, I have recommended hospitalization three times – once for a severe outbreak of psoriasis, and on two other occasions for intractably painful arterial disease of the left leg, for which he first underwent amputation of his left great toe, and later had an above-knee amputation. However, two years ago an HMO-related bureaucratic snafu occurred that seriously endangered Joseph's welfare. Once again the problem was financial or, more correctly, a question of how much money needs to be spent in order to provide good medical care. I sent the following letter to the HMO medical director, hoping to solve this issue at least for Joseph.

> *Dear Dr. ...,*
> *I am writing to you for advice and help for a patient named Joseph whom I have been following since August ... at the request of Dr. ... and his associates. The patient has been both home- and bed-bound due to a neurological problem outlined in the copies of my letters to Dr. ... that I have enclosed. Dr. ... and his colleagues do not do home visits and, since this is my specialty, I have been only too happy to assist. During the past ten months I have been instrumental in hospitalizing Joseph twice, once for control of extensive pustular psoriasis and again for amputation of an ischemic and osteomyelitic great toe.*
>
> *I visited Joseph again in June ... and the results of that examination are detailed in the accompanying letter. The most ominous finding was a progressive iron-deficiency anemia which I felt needed rapid evaluation. As you know, Dr. ..., I am boarded in internal medicine, geriatrics and gastroenterology, and spent the majority of my professional life in the latter discipline. I suggested to Dr. ... that this patient should be admitted to a hospital for colonoscopy because I felt that his wife would not be able to handle cleaning up one gallon of dirty Golytely [a pre-colonoscopic cleansing solution] from his bed.*

Dr. ... felt that this could and should be accomplished as an outpatient. It is with Dr. ...'s consent and blessing that I am writing to you as the ultimate arbiter.

In closing, I would like to have a face-to-face discussion with you about my responsibilities for your HMO's patients for whom I am officially a consultant but for whom I am really the PCP. I have many such patients whose PCPs have not seen them for years, and would appreciate your insight in handling my relationships with the patients, their referring physicians and the HMO.

Sincerely,

The medical director opted in favor of the HMO doctor. Predictably, Joseph then declined colonoscopy. His iron deficiency continues to this day. Its cause has not been found, and he requires daily iron therapy. I also never got the face-to-face meeting that I had requested.

Joseph had always been a complex individual, and had never disclosed his personal history to me. To be sure, I knew that he had been a regional (neither local nor cross-country) truck driver and that he had always loved athletics. In high school he had been on his football and baseball teams, and as a young adult he had both boxed and played baseball semi-professionally. I also knew that he had several children, but he had never told me about their lives or activities. However, one year ago I stepped into his home and, before I even had a chance to greet him, and in the presence of his wife, he opened up his life to me. He had only recently found out the seamier aspects of the story, because his wife had hidden the truth from him. His oldest son had been arrested for sexually molesting his baby daughters and for passing illegal checks. Another son had died without his knowledge, and a daughter from Joseph's first marriage had been raped by her stepfather. Joseph also told me that he had been a union "enforcer", had been in jail and had administered his share of cracked ribs and skulls to people in street fights (his wife confirmed these stories). Finally, he confided to me, with his wife standing beside us, that the "love of his life" had been a young woman with whom he had had a child but who had died years ago of breast cancer at the age of 28. Throughout this monologue, which lasted at least 40 minutes, I sat silently while Joseph talked. I thought how powerless he must have felt in the face of these catastrophic events befalling his close family members. He had always thought of himself as the man and the protector of his family. His wife had never worked, and his income alone had furnished the entire family's necessities and luxuries. Moreover, his expected union retirement income and benefits had been severely curtailed because his paralysis had occurred shortly before his retirement date. In response, I began antidepressant therapy and asked for visits from a psychiatric social worker (which the HMO approved). I also asked our social worker to visit the family. She initiated negotiations to review Joseph's benefits and increase his income. Within two months he had lost his ornery edge and become more placid and manageable, and he has remained so ever since.

Ann is a 61-year-old woman who has had multiple sclerosis for the past 20 years. She initially noted occasional episodes of staggering gait and imbalance, but chose to disregard these. Fifteen years ago, as these events became more frequent and severe, she was no longer able to ignore them and sought medical advice. The diagnosis was multiple sclerosis. The disease has primarily affected her lower extremity muscle strength and her sense of balance. Her upper body strength, vision, speech and cognition have remained intact over the past 15 years.

When Ann was diagnosed with multiple sclerosis, she was working as a loan officer at a local bank where she had started work as a teller years before. Shortly after her diagnosis, her husband deserted her with the excuse that ''I just can't handle it.'' She was left with her three children (two girls aged 20 and 18 years, and a 14-year-old boy), for whose welfare she became totally responsible. She tried to continue to work at the bank, but found that the strain of going to work and looking after her home and children without any support system was too great, and she became homebound. Her children are all college graduates, have professional jobs, and maintain a close and loving bond with her. Ann is an only child. Her mother, to whom she was close, died years ago.

Ann lives alone and spends almost all her time in bed. However, she gets out of bed daily and goes around her house checking on items by crawling across the floor. Because of her normal upper body strength, she has full bed mobility and has never had a pressure ulcer. Her son, who is also her power of attorney, visits his mother daily, does her shopping and performs errands. Ann sees her daughters every one to two weeks. Her long-term home health aide, with whom she is good friends, tends her daily for three hours and assists her in dressing and bathing, prepares her meals, does the laundry and cleans the house. Ann is continent of bowel but functionally incontinent of urine. She uses the telephone, takes her own medications and pays her own bills.

Ann has always been upbeat and an excellent conversationalist. Far from being depressed, she is funny and, like so many great comedians, pokes fun at herself without any evidence of underlying bitterness or self-pity. Whenever I arrive, some of her many friends are usually visiting her. They are always chatting merrily and graciously invite me to join in. Once, when Ann and I were alone discussing her life story, she told me "You can't dwell on the past. Always look to the future – *otherwise you go crazy!*"

Ben is a 25-year-old man who was my patient for only seven months. Two months before I met him, he had been driving a car with his girlfriend beside him and his best friend in the back seat. None of them was wearing a seat belt. Another car swerved in front of Ben's vehicle and, in order to avoid colliding with it, Ben also swerved out of his way but directly into a tree. At the last moment, Ben threw himself over his girlfriend's body to protect her. She emerged from the accident with only a few bruises, Ben's best friend was thrown from the car and immediately killed, and Ben became paraplegic. The driver of the car that Ben had tried to avoid was never identified, and drove on, probably completely unaware of the havoc in his wake.

Shortly after the accident, Ben had undergone multiple operations to repair fractures of his pelvis and spine, and was recuperating at home. He was unable to move off his back or out of bed due to stabilizing surgical pins in his pelvis, and he was in great pain that required large doses of narcotics for control. He was able to feed himself, but was dependent for changing his clothes and bathing. He was incontinent of both bowel and bladder.

When I first met Ben, he and his 47-year-old mother and primary caregiver were crying but bravely trying to hide their tears from each other. Ben's mother was a superb caregiver, and carefully maintained his nutrition with his favorite foods and by encouraging him to eat. Ben's father had died, but his mother had recently remarried. Her new husband (Ben's stepfather) had proved to be a great support and helpmate for the whole family. Ben's 27-year-old sister also stopped by twice per week. His friends, including his girlfriend, were frequent visitors. After graduating from high school, Ben had worked as a laborer at the same job for seven years. He had also been a high-school athlete, and athletic competition with his friends and neighborhood teams had remained an important part of his life until the accident. Since the accident he had felt particularly guilty about the death of his best friend, a guilt that was deepened by the fact that his friend's family had filed a wrongful death suit against him.

At my first visit, Ben's depression made such a powerful impression that I initiated antidepressant therapy as well as medications to slow down bone dissolution. One month later, I was delighted to find that Ben was actually upbeat and that his appetite had improved and he was sleeping soundly through the night. Two months after taking on his care, I arranged for transportation for removal of his surgical pins, and soon afterwards arranged for his admission to a local rehabilitation institute. I told Ben that this admission would be the start of his new life and that he could look forward to independent mobility in a wheelchair, working, marriage and even driving a car, but that this would all depend on his commitment to these goals and on hard work. During his six-week rehabilitation admission, I followed his progress by talking with his mother.

When I visited Ben shortly after his discharge, there had been a remarkable change in him. His upper body physique, which had always been sculpted, was now even larger. He was getting out of his house daily and was anxious to demonstrate to me his ability to transfer from bed to his new lightweight manual wheelchair (no power chair for him!) and scamper around the block (during his hospitalization, I had arranged for construction of a wheelchair ramp for his house). Ben's previous employer had held his job open for him, and offered to make him foreman of his warehouse. He was planning to investigate learning to drive a car using manual controls. Seven months after the accident, he was still seeing his girlfriend frequently and asked me for a prescription for sildenafil (I immediately granted his request).

At my last visit to Ben and his mother, she told me that they were going to buy a house north of Philadelphia that was within easy driving and commuting range, was all on one floor and had no steps either inside or leading up to the house. This would make the house wheelchair-friendly. I told them that I would arrange for Ben's care by a physiatrist in his new neighborhood. When we said goodbye, the three of us hugged each other tearfully. Both Ben and his mother said that they would never forget me. I shall certainly never forget them – Ben's bravery and hard work and his mother's devotion to her son.

Louis is a 28-year-old man who became quadriplegic at the C5–6 level when he dived head first into a pool at the age of 13 years. Immediately after the accident he underwent spinal fusion surgery, and several years thereafter had upper extremity tendon transplants to further develop his hand function. He has maintained the use of both thumbs and can therefore write, feed himself and use a computer keyboard. However, he is totally dependent for bathing and dressing, and is incontinent of bowel and bladder but is able to catheterize himself several times per day. He lives in a Philadelphia "wheelchair community" where all members are wheelchair bound and can each live alone in their own apartment, but require daily visits from home health aides to transfer them from bed to wheelchair to commode, to dress and bathe them, and to prepare their meals and/or feed them. In his motorized wheelchair, Louis travels to the city center via public transportation to meet friends, attend classes and see shows, and he also visits nearby supermarkets or pharmacies to shop for his daily needs. He has an ongoing friendship with a woman, with whom he has sexual relations with the help of sildenafil.

Louis was orphaned shortly after his accident, and responsibility for him passed to his paternal grandparents, with whom he is in close touch. He also has a 35-year-old brother in Florida with whom he is in constant contact. His government stipend amounts to only slightly more than 500 dollars per month, but contributions from his grandparents and brother give him a better lifestyle than most of his wheelchair-bound friends. Louis is unusually intelligent. He plays competitive chess on his computer, and he initially took college courses for credit on his computer, but has more recently traveled to a local Philadelphia university to engage in direct classroom discussion. He needs just five more courses to earn his degree, and I have no doubt that he will gain it. At one of my recent visits, he told me that he had volunteered for office work at a social service agency. After three months of volunteering, the agency's head asked him to consider working for her three days per week, eight hours per day for a salary, an offer that he promptly accepted. On non-working days he takes his university courses, reads and socializes.

Conversing with Louis is delightful. His conversational style can be serious when he is discussing local, national and international current events (about which he is well versed), or humorous and peppered with Yiddish expressions such as "Oy veh." He is particularly knowledgeable about quadriplegia and its complications. I never need to offer detailed explanations of his condition because he so thoroughly understands our conversation, including the medical vocabulary. He informed me a few months ago that he had become politically active and had become a member (by invitation) of the Pennsylvania Rehabilitation Council Committee, the group that advises the Governor and the State Board of Vocational Rehabilitation on issues regarding the handicapped (Louis would never tolerate the term 'disabled'). To do this, he travels once per month by Amtrak (these trains do not easily accommodate wheelchairs) from Philadelphia to Harrisburg, and returns home the same evening. From the train station, he takes public transportation back to his apartment and is ready for either work or school the next morning. Louis has also recently joined a new organization, Cash and Counsel, which is negotiating with government and HMOs to make funds that are ordinarily given directly to nurses and aides for handicapped patient care directly to the patients for appropriate disbursement. This would empower patients to undertake their own care, but Louis and his colleagues realize that the method for such disbursement would need to be carefully worked out.

Louis has such a strong and infectious personality that I broached with him the possibility that he might write a book about the experience of being handicapped. He replied that he didn't think he had the literary skill to accomplish this. I then said that he might consider a theatrical or acting career *à la* Christopher Reeve, and that he certainly has the personal credentials to speak for the handicapped and about their experience. For a moment his eyes glinted. Several days later, I called a nationally known theatrical school in Philadelphia and asked them to send him a brochure. I feel that with interest, devotion and hard work by Louis, and a modicum of luck, we may in a few years be watching a new theatrical personality and spokesman for the handicapped.

The care of a patient with either a congenital birth defect or a genetic disease that becomes manifest in mid-life is often a devastating blow to the entire family. In most cases the mother becomes the primary caregiver for the patient and, if her child's disease is sufficiently severe, she finds herself confined to the home, unable to socialize with other family members or peers, and unable to pursue a career. Not infrequently, the husband may desert his family if he is unable to face the responsibility or guilt of having fathered the child, or the likelihood of limitless years of child support without his wife's income (she would be unable to work because she would need to stay at home with the child). Even if the couple stay together, their marriage may be painful if they realize that the only experiences that link them revolve around their ill child. Family members other than the parents (e.g. siblings, grandparents), out of concern and love for the parents, may feel obliged to delay or alter their own life plans in order to offer assistance. However, if the cognitive abilities of the affected child or adult are sufficiently hampered, it may be difficult for anyone other than the mother to relate to him or her. For these reasons, the mother is usually the most important and reliable support for the patient with either congenital or birth defects or genetic defects that become manifest later in life.

Janice is a 50-year-old woman who was diagnosed with Huntington's chorea (HC) at the age of 36 years. The disease has an autosomal-dominant pattern of inheritance (men and women inherit the disease with equal frequency, and if the gene is inherited, the disease will definitely occur). HC usually presents in mid-life with clumsiness or spontaneous involuntary muscular movements. The disease is also associated with personality changes and, in the later stages, with dementia. The patient is eventually unable to walk and becomes bed-bound.

The onset often occurs after the age of 35 years, which usually means that the defective gene will have been passed on to a new generation. The life expectancy after onset of symptoms is around 15–20 years.

Janice's mother, now 70 years old, was married at the age of 20 and had two daughters. She and her husband divorced after 20 years because of insoluble incompatibilities. At the time of their divorce, Janice's father had been healthy. However, about seven years later he developed neurological signs of HC, and the diagnosis was confirmed by a neurologist. He subsequently died at the age of 69 years due to complications of the disease. Meanwhile the mother, who was responsible for both girls, continued to work. At the age of 36 years, Janice developed a stumbling gait accompanied by muscular jerks. The diagnosis of HC was once again confirmed. Just one year later, Janice's sister, who is 11 months younger, developed similar symptoms and she too has been diagnosed with HC. Janice had worked as a waitress and her sister was a professional drummer. Both sisters had loved to dance. Before the onset of HC, Janice had been married, but her husband left her soon after she was diagnosed. However, Janice had already had three children (two girls now aged 16 and 30 years, and a 15-year-old boy). Her sister had also had two children before she was stricken. The shadow of HC hangs over the entire younger generation, but they won't know whether they have escaped the disease for decades to come.

Janice and her sister (who is also my patient) live with their mother and Janice's 16-year-old daughter, who bears no responsibility for her mother's care. Janice's mother is the sole caregiver for both Janice and her sister. Both are bed-bound with contracted limbs and are highly demented, and they both require tube feeding. Although Janice is relatively quiet unless she is handled or disturbed, her sister yells throughout the day and night without any apparent provocation. The mother's only assistance comes from her mother (Janice's grandmother), who is now 90 years old and too infirm to be of substantial help. The mother is always at home tending her daughters. She only gets out of the house every other week to attend church.

Despite the mother's onerous duties, she has a remarkably cheerful and upbeat attitude. She attributes this to her strong religious faith and her daily devotional readings. This faith and trust in God is pervasive in the black community. Time and again I have seen it bolster frail people with agonizing burdens. However, I would personally have hoped that she might have had the same faith without this reason to test it.

Laura is a 30-year-old woman with both cerebral palsy and severe mental retardation. She also has a medically controlled petit-mal seizure disorder and prominent gastroesophageal reflux with recurrent episodes of aspiration pneumonia. These have been so severe that she recently underwent surgical repair of her gastroesophageal sphincter mechanism. Laura also has chronic idiopathic intestinal pseudo-obstruction. Because of this, she requires both a jejunostomy tube through which she is fed a special liquid diet directly into the small intestine, and a gastrostomy tube which serves as a decompression site should food back up. Laura shows no awareness of, meaningful contact with or response to her surroundings. She grunts or screams unintelligibly and thrashes about on her bed without any apparent provocation. Of course she is bed-bound and totally dependent on her mother for all her care.

Laura's mother is a 54-year-old ICU registered nurse, the cream of her profession. She grew up in Charleston, South Carolina, and developed a love for reading early in life. Regarded by her peers and family as a "bookworm", she graduated with honors from high school at the age of 16 years, and then went to college in her home town to study nursing. After graduating with her RN degree, she worked in med–surg nursing but then gravitated to the ICU. She married in college and had four children, of whom Laura is the youngest. Her three sons are 37, 35 and 31 years old. All of the sons are married with children and have good government administrative jobs. They are also all close to her and live in Philadelphia. The middle son occasionally comes to help out. However, her husband left the family soon after Laura was born, moved across the country and maintains contact with his three sons but not with his wife, nor does he ever ask about his daughter.

Unlike many other women in similar situations, Laura's mother works full-time on the 11–7 (night) shift in the ICU. She comes home in the morning and goes straight to bed. On awakening in the afternoon, she immediately attends to Laura (e.g. by administering her medicines and feedings, bathing her, and cleaning and changing her) and then does the shopping, the laundry and the house cleaning and pays the bills. She has some help from her 23-year-old niece, but the majority of the routine and all of the professional responsibility rests with her. Laura's mother has no free time for socializing. All of her socializing occurs on her job or with her family members. She spends her minimal spare time reading novels, professional journals or devotional literature (again, the religious connection). She sees no exit from her present life.

Summation

Pediatricians like to say that their patients are not just small adults. Likewise, the homebound have their own medical and social problems that are not discernible from study of healthy ambulatory or independent adults. My elderly patients have a particularly keenly pervasive *sense of loss*, because they have lost so many friends and family members, their professional identities, and particularly their physical and mental attributes, which they had always taken for granted.

Home visits provide a front-line means of protecting the health of our homebound, shoring up their capabilities for independence and simultaneously keeping them out of emergency rooms, hospitals and nursing homes, all of which are extremely expensive. This responsibility should ideally be allocated to mature, experienced clinicians with long experience in the management of patients with *multiple chronic diseases*. A reservoir of such physicians exists among recently retired doctors. Many of our older physicians, who were trained in a different age (and perhaps with different value systems), are demoralized for a variety of reasons, including the ''hassle factor'' from government, HMOs and insurance companies, the extraordinary rise in malpractice insurance premiums, and the loosening of personal ties to patients promoted by HMOs. I have talked to many retired physicians who sorely miss patient care, but who would rather not return to the practice of medicine now, due to the above factors.

However, I believe that we can reclaim these retired physicians' services *and their professional enthusiasm* by asking them to recommit themselves, either full-time or part-time, to the care of the homebound, a population to which any of us may some day belong. To accomplish this, we would need at the very least a reduction in malpractice insurance premiums for these retired or semi-retired physicians, a brief brush-up course in the physiology and special problems of the homebound, adequate secretarial and social service support, and a recognition both verbally and by financial recompense that appropriate home visits are valuable. The enormous profits gained from this program would include:

1 the gratitude of an otherwise neglected but very deserving segment of our society

2 rejuvenation of interest by many physicians in the most basic principles of our profession that are so well expressed in the Hippocratic Oath

3 cost savings of dollars spent on well-meaning but often misguided efforts to provide health care by sending these patients to an emergency room, hospitalizing them or placing them in nursing homes. These patients' interests could be better met by more efficient home visits and appropriate home care or hospice care.

My partner and I work 8 to 12 hours per day. However, only about 60% of our time is spent in face-to-face contact with patients. The remainder of our working day is spent in paperwork and making telephone calls to nurses, physical, occupational and speech therapists, pharmacists, social workers and psychologists, hospital staff and referring physicians, and to patients and their caregivers, with whom we spend much time teaching, cajoling, counseling and consoling. This behind-the-scenes activity, which is at least as important to our mission as patient confrontation and physical contact, is not reimbursable by Medicare or insurance agencies. Few recent graduates of internal medicine or family practice residency training programs will be interested in such a career. These young doctors are often already saddled with formidable educational debt, and many of them are married with children. Upon completion of their residency programs, they would sooner gravitate to subspecialty fellowship programs that offer either a larger income, a more stress-free lifestyle, or both.

Home visits are certainly not a panacea for medical patients in general. However, they are the method of choice for delivering basic and preventive care to people who would not otherwise receive such care. This population has been described as using huge amounts of financial resources at advanced stages in their disease processes. From a purely monetary standpoint, our health system would save large sums that could be well spent in other areas of health care delivery. Mobilization and training of physicians for this project could be coordinated through organizations such as the American Medical Association, the American College of Physicians, the American Academy of Family Practice, the American Geriatrics Society and the American Academy of Home Care Physicians. Administration could occur through the Centers for Medicare and Medicaid Services under the Department of Health and Human Services. The need is there – the time is now.

Glossary

ACE (angiotensin-converting enzyme) inhibitors A class of medications that are used to treat hypertension and congestive heart failure.

Achalasia A neuromuscular disorder of the esophagus that results in difficulty swallowing, weight loss, and recurrent pneumonia due to aspiration.

Alzheimer's disease A gradually progressive disease of the brain that is the commonest cause of dementia in the United States today.

Angina A syndrome manifested primarily by chest pain, but also by sweating or shortness of breath on exertion or even at rest, often signifying decreased blood flow to the cardiac muscle.

Angiography Imaging methods used for visualization of the vascular system.

Aortic stenosis Obstruction of the aortic valve – that is, the heart valve situated between the left ventricle and the aorta (the main artery of the body).

Aphasia Impairment of the ability to express oneself in or to comprehend spoken or written language, due to damage to certain brain centers.

Apnea Cessation of breathing.

Arteriosclerotic heart disease Heart disease caused by obstruction of coronary vessels.

Atrial fibrillation An abnormal heart rhythm caused by disordered conduction of electrical impulses from the atria to the ventricles, resulting in an irregular heart beat. The condition predisposes to strokes.

Bariatric Referring to weight reduction, usually of large magnitude.

Beta-blockers A class of medications that are used to treat hypertension, congestive heart failure, heart attacks and angina, and to control certain cardiac arrhythmias.

Capitation The practice of some health maintenance organizations of awarding a low monthly fee per patient to physicians to cover their total health care. This is only advantageous to the physician if he or she has a large patient population that is essentially healthy.

Cellulitis Diffuse inflammation of soft or connective tissue (usually skin), due to infection.

Chronic idiopathic intestinal pseudo-obstruction An uncommon neuromuscular disorder of the gastrointestinal tract that results in poor propulsion of intestinal contents and poor absorption of nutrients.

Chronic ulcerative colitis An inflammatory colonic disease involving the innermost layers of the colon. Features of the disease may affect extra-colonic tissues such as the joints, skin, eyes and liver.

Congestive heart failure A group of conditions that result in inability of the heart to pump as much blood as the body requires.

Contracture Fixed high resistance to passive stretch of muscles adjacent to a joint, caused by replacement of the joint's supporting tissues with fibrous tissue.

Dementia Organic loss of intellectual function or, more simply, the ability to think. This is commonly divided into various domains, such as memory, calculation, facility with language, abstract reasoning, executive ability, etc.

Diuresis Increased excretion of urine.

Dyspnea Shortness of breath.

Echocardiogram An ultrasonographic procedure that can provide information about cardiac structure and function.

Emphysema A chronic lung disease associated with increased lung volume due to enlargement of the air sacs through which gas exchange is effected. It is commonly but not necessarily associated with tobacco smoking.

Encephalopathy   Any degenerative disease of the brain.

Endocarditis   Inflammation of the innermost lining of the heart, most commonly involving a heart valve.

Endoscopy   Visual inspection of any body cavity by means of a hollow or fiberoptic tube.

Fistula   An abnormal (or occasionally a surgically created) connection between two hollow organs, or between a hollow organ and the skin surface.

Formulary   A list of medications provided by a hospital or HMO.

Gastroesophageal reflux   Regurgitation of gastric acid through an incompetent lower esophageal protective mechanism (sphincter) into the esophagus, often causing heartburn and occasionally causing cough, bleeding and ulceration.

Gastroesophageal sphincter   The high-pressure zone in the lower esophagus that normally (except during vomiting or belching) prevents regurgitation of gastric contents back into the esophagus.

Gastrostomy   The surgical or endoscopic creation of an opening from the abdominal wall into the stomach.

Gerichair   A frame chair with wheels and a moveable tray suitable for maintaining a patient in position and for serving meals.

Glaucoma   A group of eye diseases that are characterized by increased pressure within the globe and which, if untreated, result in blindness.

Hemangioma   A tumor formed from vascular tissue.

Hemiparesis   Paralysis of one side of the body.

Hemochromatosis   A disease in which the body absorbs and stores excessive amounts of iron, which is deposited in and damages various organs, including the liver, pancreas, heart and joints.

Hemodialysis   The practice of intermittently removing by machine toxins from the blood of patients with chronic kidney failure, or acutely from patients with acute kidney failure or who have ingested poisons or excessive medication.

Histologically   Referring to confirmation by biopsy and microscopic proof.

HMO (health maintenance organization)   An organization that endeavors to control the cost of medical care by means which include capitation, and controlled access to consultants and special procedures.

Hypoglycemic   Referring to low blood sugar.

Jejunostomy   The surgical or endoscopic creation of an opening between the jejunum (the second portion of the small intestine) and the abdominal wall.

Medicaid   Individual state-administered organizations which, in conjunction with the federal government, administer funds for medical support of the poor.

Medicare   US government organization that administers medical support funds to the elderly and other special populations, such as patients with disabling mental illness or who are on hemodialysis, etc.

Metastasis   Spread of cancer to distant sites.

Mitral valve   The heart valve situated between the left atrium and the left ventricle.

MMSE (Mini Mental State Examination)   A 30-point test for dementia, that is easily and rapidly administered, reproducible, and which addresses several domains of dementia. It is the most commonly used test for dementia.

Morbidity and Mortality Committee   A Committee formed by physicians to formally investigate and discuss adverse incidents and deaths.

Multiple sclerosis   A neurological disease characterized by patchy loss of nerve sheaths (myelin) throughout the central nervous system, and associated with weakness, incoordination, numbness, and speech and visual problems.

Myocardial infarction   Heart attack.

Neurogenic pain   Pain caused by damage to the central or peripheral nervous system. Chronic neurogenic pain is often resistant to multiple medical therapies.

Neuropsychiatric examination   The "gold standard" for detecting dementia. It can accurately discriminate depression from dementia, and it can detect dementia long before other commonly used tests for dementia. It must be administered by a trained neuropsychologist.

Osteoarthritis   Degenerative joint disease occurring chiefly in older people, particularly but not necessarily affecting the weight-bearing joints, and accompanied by pain and stiffness in these joints.

Osteopenia   Any decrease in bone mass below normal levels.

Paraplegia   Paralysis of the lower limbs, usually due to trauma to the low spinal cord, and often associated with bowel and bladder paralysis.

Pathological fracture   Fracture due to trauma of bone weakened by cancer invasion or other causes.

Peripheral arterial disease   Narrowing of arteries to the lower extremities, commonly causing pain during walking or, when the disease is more severe, even at rest. Extreme disease may result in necrosis (death) of the toes, feet or legs.

Physiology   The science pertaining to understanding of the functions of the living organism.

Platform walker   An assistive device for walking, in which the patient rests his or her forearms on a platform and guides the walker's direction. It is designed for patients whose hand grip is insufficiently strong to grasp the rails of a standard walker.

Polymyalgia rheumatica   A rheumatoid-type disease of muscles of the elderly, characterized by muscle pain in the hip and shoulder girdles.

Pressure ulcer   Skin breakdown due to prolonged pressure to its vascular supply by the surface on which the patient is resting.

Primary caregiver   The person who is primarily responsible for maintaining the patient's physical, psychological and economic welfare.

Primary thrombocytosis   An increased number of platelets in the peripheral blood, of unknown cause.

Psoriasis   A chronic, recurrent, hereditary, immunological skin disease that may also affect the joints.

Pulmonary emboli   Blood clots originating in the legs or pelvis or, less commonly, the right side of the heart and carried to the pulmonary artery, where they obstruct blood flow to the lungs.

Pyrosis   Heartburn.

Quadriplegia   Paralysis of all four limbs.

Rheumatoid arthritis   A chronic progressive immunological systemic disease affecting primarily the joints, but many other parts of the body as well.

Spina bifida   A developmental anomaly characterized by defective closure of the bony encasement of the spinal cord, through which the cord and its covering membrane may or may not protrude.

Ureteroenterostomy   A surgical connection between the urinary and gastrointestinal systems that causes urine to empty into a bag attached to the abdominal wall.